FOREWORD

From Sir Robert Balchin,
Director General 1984-1990,
Founder of The Three Cross Award.

1, Grosvenor Crescent
London SW1X 7EF

Dear Colleague,

It is now ten years since the first edition of *Emergency Aid in Schools* was published. I am thankful that during the past decade more and more teachers have become aware of the need for first aid skills and I believe that this little book, now read by several hundred thousand teachers, has contributed to that awareness.

Just occasionally comes the moment dreaded by all of us who look after young people, instead of the usual minor grazes and bruises, we are faced with a severe accident. A child might be drowning or be bleeding profusely, a staff member may have suffered a heart attack, and we have to cope.

It is a fearful responsibility and yet there are a few simple procedures that anyone can learn and which, if applied correctly during the first minutes after the accident, could mean the difference between life and death.

These procedures, called Emergency Aid, are detailed in this book with examples of accidents that have actually happened in schools. Do remember, however, that although this book will equip you with many of the skills that you need in an emergency, it is no substitute for a course in First Aid. Such a course, based on this book, need not take more than a few hours and can be arranged at your school. Full details can be found on page 67.

Please keep this book where you teach so that you can refer to it easily and please re-read it regularly; you never know, one of your pupils might have cause to thank you for it someday!

I am grateful to you for taking an interest in First Aid.

Yours very sincerely,

Robert Balchin

CONTENTS

HOW TO USE THIS BOOK

Emergency Aid in Schools has been carefully structured to enable teachers to use it in three ways:

1 As a form of basic instruction about Emergency Aid

2 As an aide-memoire; for 'refresher training'

3 As a reference book in an emergency

The opening chapter *'Emergency action'* introduces the essential techniques and procedures which should be followed in an emergency.

Chapters 2 to 8 provide:

* **Essential information** on the specific area covered in the chapter
* **Step-by-step techniques** giving basic instruction about Emergency Aid
* **Scenarios** suggesting different school contexts in which emergencies may occur; followed by emergency procedures which help to test and reinforce what has been learned in the step-by-step techniques

The Emergency index on page 74 allows teachers to locate instantly the correct procedures to follow in an emergency.

It is hoped that having read the book you will be motivated to undertake First Aid training: details of courses run by St. John Ambulance are on page 67.

Note

Most Emergency Aid principles and procedures apply equally to both children and adults. However, sometimes the procedure may vary slightly because of the differing needs of a child's smaller, younger body. In judging whether to use adult or child procedure, the best criterion to use is the size of the child. Physical stature is the key and the first aider will have to use his or her commonsense. If there is any doubt, use the procedures described for a child.

In this book adult techniques are described with the modifications required for handling a child casualty shown in a separate box or on a separate page.

Resuscitation and choking procedures for babies are different and have not been included because you will not need them in school. You can become competent in these procedures by joining a St. John Ambulance Lifesaver for Babies and Children course, lasting four hours.

In most cases the accidents that occur in a school are minor and the injuries can be easily treated. On those infrequent occasions when a serious accident occurs, it is essential that you know when medical assistance must be summoned and what you can do whilst waiting for that help to arrive. This book is designed to help you to learn some of the procedures that are needed when giving Emergency Aid.

Better still, enrol in a First Aid training course – the confidence which can be provided only by practice is invaluable.

Remember to be careful of your own personal safety.

THE EMERGENCY PROCEDURE

Assess the situation
Keep calm and find out what has happened as quickly as you can.

Make safe
Is the casualty in danger? Are other colleagues and pupils safe? Take action to protect them, but do not put yourself at risk. Do not try to do too much yourself.

Emergency Aid
Assess the casualty's condition and take appropriate action. (To do this you will need to read the rest of this book and preferably get further training.)

Get Help
Obtain qualified help as early as you can and use colleagues and pupils to provide assistance.

Aftermath
Prepare yourself to make a concise hand-over to the ambulance crew. Organise the care of other pupils and staff who may be distressed. Ensure that the scene is cleared up and restock your kit if you have used any. Report the incident using your school's normal procedure.

When life is at risk
The vast majority of emergency situations you will have to deal with at school will not endanger life. However, it is essential that you are prepared for an incident where a life may be at risk.

Since the rapid application of the correct Emergency Aid can save lives, it is essential that you know how to assess a casualty's condition quickly. With this in mind, please read this opening section as carefully as you can.

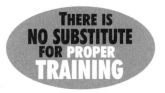

Emergency Aid in school ———
Whatever you may be feeling when an emergency occurs at school, stay calm.
If you know how to provide Emergency Aid it is important that you tell the casualty what you are intending to do. Continue to talk in a reassuring way while you are giving treatment.

ASSESSING THE CASUALTY

When you have assessed the situation at the scene of the incident at school, you can begin to deal with the sick or injured casualty.

Although there may be obvious injuries, your first step is to make an urgent assessment solely for life threatening priorities, the so-called "Initial Assessment".
This sequence is:

> **Danger**
> **Response**
> **Airway**
> **Breathing**
> **Circulation**
>
> or **D.R.A.B.C.**

Once you have cleared any danger, check response in order to decide if the casualty is unconscious, as an unconscious casualty must always be given immediate Emergency Aid. To check this, shout "Can you hear me?" or "Open your eyes".
Shake the casualty's shoulders carefully.

If the casualty is conscious, is breathing and has a pulse, check for bleeding, treat as appropriate and get help if necessary.

If there is no response, the casualty is unconscious and you should follow the resuscitation sequence.

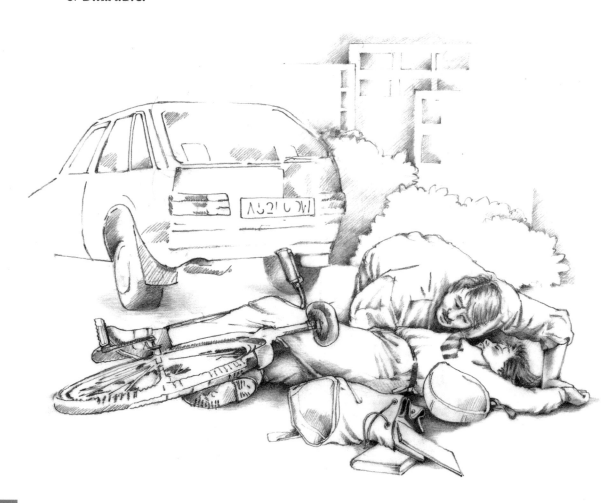

THE RESUSCITATION SEQUENCE

A Clear and open airway

In an unconscious casualty, the tongue may fall to the back of the throat, blocking the air passage (airway).

1 Place two fingers under the point of the casualty's chin.
2 Place your other hand on the casualty's forehead.
3 At the same time, lift the jaw and tilt the head back.

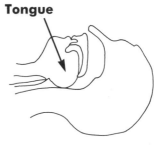

Blocked airway

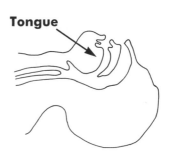

Open airway

B Check breathing

Put your ear close to the casualty's mouth:
1 Look for chest movements.
2 Listen to sounds of breathing.
3 Feel for breath on your cheek.

Do this for at least ten seconds before deciding whether casualty is breathing or not.
You must maintain chin lift throughout this procedure to keep the airway open.

NOTE
If the casualty is breathing, place him in the recovery position (see page 8) then check circulation.

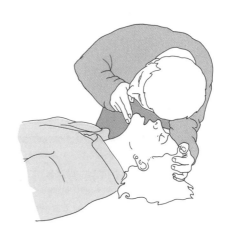

C Check circulation

Check the carotid pulse:
1 Locate the carotid pulse in the hollow between the voice box and the main muscle of the neck.
2 Feel the pulse by pressing your finger tips gently on the artery. Do not use your thumb.
3 Check for up to ten seconds before deciding that there is no heartbeat.

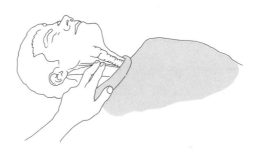

Emergency Aid for an adult

Unconscious, is breathing

- Place in recovery position.
- Check pulse.
- Check for severe bleeding.
- Treat as appropriate.
- Call for help.

Unconscious, not breathing

- Not due to injury or drowning ⇨ go for help immediately. Reassess DRAB and then continue sequence.
- Due to injury or drowning ⇨ complete one minute of ventilation or CPR (as appropriate) then go for help. Reassess DRAB and then continue sequence.

- Give two breaths of mouth-to-mouth ventilation.
- Check pulse.

Pulse present

- Give ten breaths of mouth-to-mouth ventilation (1 minute).
- Check pulse.
- Continue to give mouth-to-mouth ventilations, checking for pulse after every 10 breaths.

Pulse absent

- Apply CPR continuously (15 chest compressions to 2 mouth-to-mouth ventilations) until help arrives.

MOUTH-TO-MOUTH VENTILATION (ADULT)

1 Look for obvious obstruction in the mouth and quickly remove it.
2 Open the airway (see page 10).
3 Pinch the casualty's nostrils together. Take a deep breath.
4 Place your lips around the casualty's mouth. Blow into the casualty's mouth until the chest rises. Take about two seconds for full inflation.
5 Remove your lips, allowing the chest to fall completely. Take another breath whilst this is happening.
6 Repeat stages 4 and 5 as per sequence above.

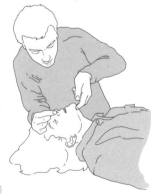
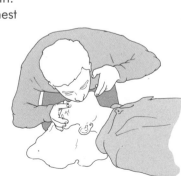

Chest compressions together with mouth-to-mouth ventilation (Adult).

Chest compressions together with mouth-to-mouth ventilation (adult). This is the sequence known as **CPR** (cardio pulmonary resuscitation).

Having carried out the DRABC assessment and found that the casualty is not breathing, given 2 breaths and checked the pulse:

1 If there is no pulse, locate the correct hand position:

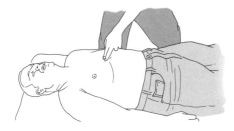

- find the point where the lower ribs meet the breastbone and keep two fingers of one hand there.

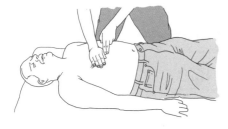

- slide the heel of the other hand down the breastbone to meet your fingers.

2 Place the heel of the first hand on top of the other and lock the fingers together.

3 Kneel so that your shoulders are directly above the casualty's breastbone. Keeping your arms straight, press the breastbone down about 4 – 5cm (1$\frac{1}{2}$ – 2″).

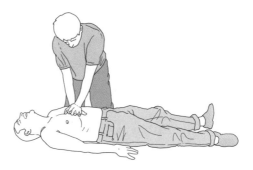

4 Release pressure, keeping your hands in place.

5 Repeat compression 15 times, aiming at a rate of 100 per minute.

6 Give two breaths of mouth-to-mouth ventilation.

7 Continue resuscitation. 15 compressions to two breaths until help arrives.

8 Only if the casualty's colour improves, check the pulse. If the pulse is present, stop the chest compressions and continue to ventilate if necessary.

See page 4 for when to call an ambulance.

///// DO NOT /////

- Use chest compression on either a child or an adult if there is a pulse, however weak.

Emergency Aid for a child

Unconscious, is breathing

- Place in recovery position.
- Check pulse.
- Check for severe bleeding.
- Treat as appropriate
- Call for help.

Unconscious, not breathing

- Give five breaths of mouth-to-mouth ventilation.
- Check carotid pulse.

Pulse present

- Give twenty breaths of mouth-to-mouth ventilation.
- If the child is small enough, carry him to the telephone and dial 999 for an ambulance.
- If you have left the child to dial 999, on your return, quickly reassess DRABC.
- Continue to give mouth-to-mouth ventilation until help arrives (check pulse every twenty breaths).

Pulse absent

- Give mouth-to-mouth ventilations and chest compressions for one minute.
- If the child is small enough, carry him to the telephone and dial 999 for an ambulance.
- If you have left the child to dial 999, on your return quickly reassess the DRABC.
- Continue to give chest compressions and mouth-to-mouth ventilations until help arrives.

NB: *When reassessing DRABC, include 5 breaths if breathing is absent before checking pulse.*

MOUTH-TO-MOUTH VENTILATION (CHILD)

1 Open the airway (see page 10).
2 Pinch the casualty's nostrils together.
3 Place your lips around the casualty's mouth, blow gently until the chest rises.
4 As the chest rises, remove your lips allowing the chest to fall completely.
5 Repeat stages 3 and 4 as per sequence above.

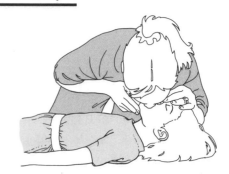

Chest compressions together with mouth-to-mouth ventilation (Child).

This is similar to adult **CPR** but with some minor variations.

Having carried out the DRABC assessment and found that the casualty is not breathing, given 2 breaths and checked the pulse:

1 If there is no pulse, locate the correct hand position:
- Find the point where the lower ribs meet the breast-bone and keep two fingers of one hand there.

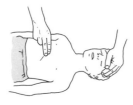

- Slide the heel of the other hand down the breast-bone to meet your fingers.

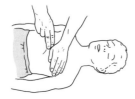

2 Use the heel of that <u>one hand</u> and press down to a third of the depth of the chest.

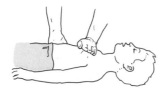

3 Release the pressure, keeping your hand in place.

4 Press <u>five</u> times at the rate of 100 compressions per minute.

5 After five compressions, blow gently into the lungs <u>once</u>.

6 Continue this process for one minute.

7 If the child is small enough, carry him to the telephone and dial 999 for an ambulance.

8 If you have left the child to dial 999, on your return quickly reassess the DRABC.

9 Continue resuscitation five compressions to one breath until the ambulance arrives.

10 Only if the casualty's colour improves check the pulse. If the pulse is present stop chest compressions and continue to ventilate if necessary.

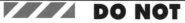 **DO NOT**
- Use chest compression on either a child or an adult if there is a pulse, however weak.

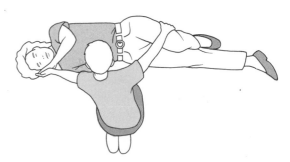

THE RECOVERY POSITION

An unconscious casualty who is breathing should always be placed in the recovery position in order to prevent the tongue from blocking the throat and to allow drainage of liquids. The following step-by-step technique assumes the casualty is lying on her back from the start. Remove spectacles and any bulky objects from the casualty's pockets if there is time.

3 With your other hand, grasp the outside of the thigh furthest away from you.
Pull the knee up, keeping the foot flat on the ground.

4 Keeping her hand pressed against her cheek, pull on the thigh to roll the casualty towards you.

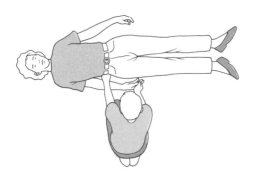

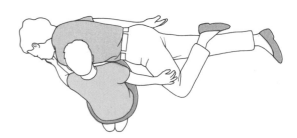

1 Straighten legs and ensure airway is open. Place arm nearest you under her upper thigh with the palm of the hand facing upwards.

2 Bring the other arm across the chest. Hold the hand, palm outward, against the casualty's nearest cheek.

5 Move upper leg, if necessary, so that hip and knee are at right-angles.

6 Ease the chin forward to keep the airway open, adjusting the hand under the cheek if necessary.

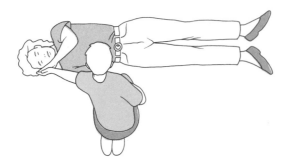

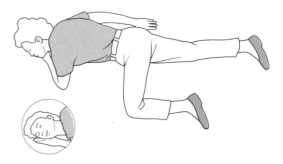

7 Adjust the lower arm so that the casualty is not lying on it. Make sure the hand is still positioned with the palm upwards.

FIRST AID HYGIENE, HIV AND HEPATITIS B

These are both viral infections that can be spread by blood to blood contact. With a little thought and pre-planning the risk of infection can be minimised.

- All blood can be a potential hazard to the first aider so avoid unnecessary unprotected contact.
- Cover any wounds or open sores you may have with a waterproof dressing.
- The use of good quality disposable latex gloves is strongly recommended.
- Good handwashing prior to treating minor wounds will protect the casualty from infection.
- Washing your hands prior to taking off contaminated gloves and again afterwards, will provide you with protection from infection.
- Blood will not pose a problem on your undamaged skin, but to minimise risk, wash off any blood as soon as possible with soap and water. If the eye or mouth or damaged skin is infected, then seek medical advice.
- Dispose of any contaminated dressings etc into yellow clinical waste sacks. These should then be incinerated.

- Clean up blood spills using an appropriate product (eg bleach granules) according to instructions. If not available, then use absorbent paper towels and bleach. Leave in place for 30 minutes. After this has been cleared, the area should be dried and waste matter disposed of in yellow sacks for incineration.

NB: *Care must be taken to ensure adequate ventilation when using the above products. Gloves should be worn when cleaning blood spillage.*

No evidence has been shown that HIV is spread by mouth-to-mouth resuscitation. If you are at all worried, then the use of a simple face shield or mask will provide protection.
The lack of shields, gloves, etc should not deter any first aider from providing assistance at the scene if an accident.
Contaminated needles are a particular risk, so great care must be taken when dealing with them. Disposal must be in a recognised sharps box.

A SCHOOL FIRST AID KIT

The qualified First Aider in a school may be responsible for replacing any items that have been used from the First Aid Kit. Listed below are the recommendation of contents that are published in the Health and Safety Commission's Code of Practice.

These are:

Guidance card	1
Individual wrapped sterile adhesive dressings	20
Sterile eye pads, with attachment	2
Triangular bandages	6
Safety pins	6

Medium sized sterile unmedicated dressings	6
Large sterile unmedicated dressings	6
Extra large sterile unmedicated dressings	3

Disposable gloves, aprons and plastic bags should also be available.

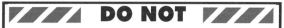

DO NOT

- keep medications such as pills or antiseptic in a First Aid kit

ESSENTIAL INFORMATION

Every cell in our bodies needs oxygen. When we breathe in, the oxygen in the air travels down the airway to the lungs. From here it enters the blood, which is then pumped around the body by the heart. When we breathe out, carbon dioxide and unused oxygen are expelled.

The process of breathing is controlled by the respiratory centre in the brain.

A disturbance of the breathing process may prevent oxygen being supplied to the brain. If the oxygen supply to the brain ceases, cells begin to die after only three minutes.

> If someone is not breathing, speed is vital. You need to start getting oxygen to the casualty's brain immediately.

Potential causes of lack of oxygen in the blood

- There may not be enough oxygen in the air being breathed in because of smoke or fumes.
- The nose, mouth or airway may be blocked.
- The blood may be poisoned, e.g. by carbon monoxide, so that it cannot carry oxygen.
- The chest wall may be crushed or injured.
- The lungs may not be working properly e.g. collapsed lung or pneumonia.

Airway

In a conscious casualty, the airway can be blocked by food, vomit, by an object or by the throat swelling after injury.

In an unconscious casualty, the tongue may fall to the back of the throat, blocking the air passage.

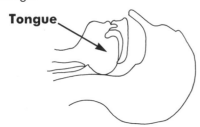

Tongue

Blocked airway

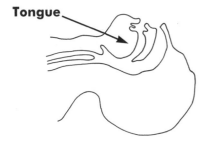

Tongue

Open airway

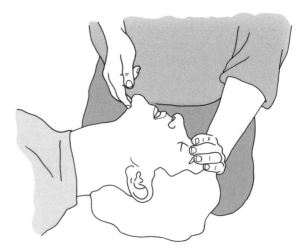

Open the airway by:
- lifting the tongue away from the air passage.

To do this:
- place two fingers under the point of the casualty's jaw.
- place your other hand on the casualty's forehead.
- at the same time, lift the jaw and tilt the head back.

Breathing

To check breathing, put your ear close to the casualty's mouth:

* Look for chest movements.
* Listen to sounds of breathing.
* Feel for breath on your cheek.

Do this for at least ten seconds before deciding whether casualty is breathing or not.

For the full resuscitation sequence, see page 3.

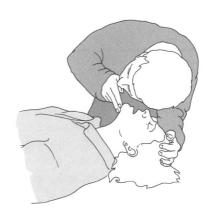

MOUTH-TO-MOUTH VENTILATION

1 With the casualty lying on the back, first remove any obvious obstruction.

2 Open the airway by lifting the chin and tilting the head back (see opposite).

3 Pinch the casualty's nostrils together. Take a deep breath.

4 Place your lips around the casualty's mouth. Blow into the casualty's mouth until the chest rises.

5 Remove your lips, allowing the chest to fall. Take another breath.

6 Repeat stages 3, 4 and 5 as appropriate

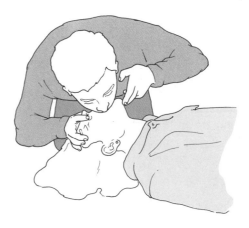

NOTE

In situations such as rescue from water, or where mouth injuries make a good seal impossible, mouth-to-nose ventilation may be more effective. To do this lift the chin, ensure the casualty's mouth and lips are sealed, form a tight seal around her nose and blow. Let the expired breath come out through the mouth.

General rules for when casualty is not breathing

* Act quickly.
* Follow the resuscitation sequence: open the airway; check breathing; check circulation.
* Be prepared to apply mouth-to-mouth ventilation until professional help arrives.

CHOKING

Recognition
- difficulty in speaking
- difficulty in breathing
- casualty may go red and then blue in the face
- casualty may point at or grasp their throat

Aims of treatment
- remove whatever is obstructing the airway
- restore normal breathing

TREATMENT

1 Reassure casualty, bend him forward with the head lower than the chest. Slap up to five times between the shoulder blades. See if you can now remove the obstruction.
2 If this is unsuccessful, try up to five abdominal thrusts. Stand behind the casualty, interlock your hands below his rib cage, then pull sharply inward and upwards.
3 Continue alternating five back slaps and five abdominal thrusts until the obstruction clears.

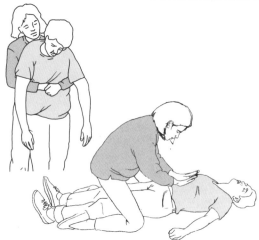

4 If the casualty becomes unconscious, check breathing (see page 4).

If not breathing:
- turn on one side and give up to five slaps between the shoulder blades. See if you can now remove the obstruction.
- if these are unsuccessful, kneel astride the casualty and give up to five abdominal thrusts.
- if now breathing normally, place in recovery position (see page 8) and call an ambulance.
If still not breathing, apply mouth-to-mouth ventilation (see page 4).

TREATMENT OF A CHILD

1 Encourage the child to cough if possible. Look in the mouth and remove any visible and easily grasped object. DO NOT probe blindly.
2 Bend her forward, so that her head is lower than her chest. Give up to five firm slaps between the shoulder blades.
3 If this does not work, stand or kneel behind the child. Make a fist and place it against her lower breastbone. Grasp it with your other hand. Press into the chest with a quick inward thrust (chest thrust) up to five times.
4 If unsuccessful, give up to another five back slaps.
5 If this does not work, give abdominal thrusts as you would to an adult. Repeat up to five times.
6 If this does not work, dial 999. Continue repeating the sequence: back slaps, chest thrusts, back slaps, abdominal thrusts.

If breathing stops at any time, apply mouth-to-mouth ventilation (see page 6) and call an ambulance.

///// DO NOT /////

- Try to remove an obstruction from a child's mouth if there is ANY danger that you might push it down the throat.
- Touch the back of a young child's throat.

SCENARIO

A young child is choking on a small piece of a construction toy.

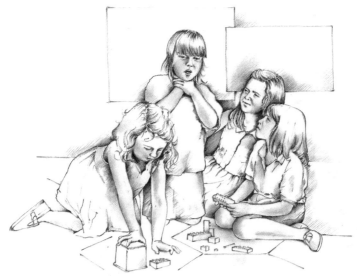

A If you can see the object in the child's mouth but it is near the back of the throat, would you remove it with your fingers?

B In what position do you put the child to start Emergency Aid?

Assess

The girl is in considerable distress and is finding it difficult to breathe.

Make safe

Do not waste time, but if someone is at hand, call him or her to look after the other children while you treat the casualty.

Get Help

If the Emergency Aid procedures do not work, dial 999.

Aftermath

Follow normal procedures for reporting an accident.

Emergency Aid

- Look in the child's mouth. If there is no danger of pushing the object down her throat, try to remove it with your fingers.
- See if she can cough up the object.
- Place her over your knees, head down. Slap up to five times between the shoulder blades.
- If this does not work:
  - stand or kneel behind the child and give up to five chest thrusts (see page 12).
  - if unsuccessful, give up to another five back slaps.
  - If this does not work, give up to five abdominal thrusts (see page 12).
- If this still does not work, dial 999. Continue repeating the sequence: back slaps, chest thrusts, back slaps, abdominal thrusts.

If breathing stops at any time, apply mouth-to-mouth ventilation (see page 6).

ASTHMA

This can be a very distressing condition. In an asthma attack the muscles of the air passages go into spasm, making breathing out particularly difficult. An attack may be triggered by an allergy or nervous tension. People who suffer from asthma usually know how to cope with an attack and are likely to carry medication which dilates the air passages.

Recognition
- difficulty in breathing, especially breathing out
- wheeziness when breathing out
- blueness of the skin
- distress and anxiety

In a severe attack, the effort of breathing may be so great that the casualty becomes exhausted, losing consciousness.

Aims of treatment
- make breathing easier
- obtain medical aid if attack is severe

TREATMENT

1 Reassure casualty to reduce anxiety.
2 Make sure the casualty sits down, leaning slightly forward on a table or some other support.

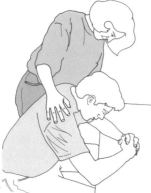

3 Ensure a plentiful supply of fresh air.
4 Find out if the casualty has medication and encourage him or her to use it. This is most likely to be a 'puffer' aerosol. On no account should somebody else's medication be used.
5 If the casualty stops breathing commence the resuscitation sequence (page 3).

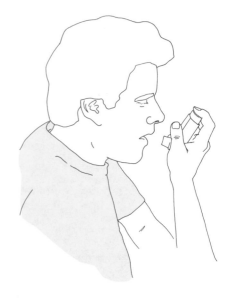

Dial 999 for an ambulance:
- if the casualty has not had an asthma attack before.
- OR if the medication fails to improve the breathing.
- OR if the casualty is in great distress.

Monitor breathing and pulse every ten minutes.

SCENARIO

A girl suffers an asthma attack during a Maths lesson.

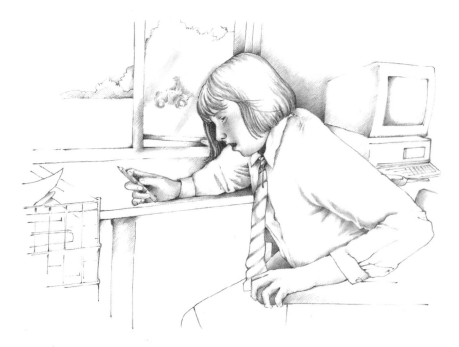

A How do you recognise an asthma attack?

B What should you do if this is the girl's first asthma attack?

Assess

The girl's breathing is laboured. She is obviously in considerable distress.

Make safe

Ensure a good supply of fresh air, reassuring her all the time.

Get Help

If it is the first attack, does not respond to medication or is prolonged, dial 999 for an ambulance.

Aftermath

Tell the girl's parents about the attack, even if it is mild. Encourage them to inform her GP.

Emergency Aid

- Sit her down at a table or desk, so that she leans slightly forward.
- Find out if the girl carries medication for asthma.
- Encourage her to use the medication.
- If she does not carry medication or if the medication fails to have an effect, call an ambulance.
- Monitor breathing and pulse every ten minutes.

UNCONSCIOUS CASUALTY – DROWNING

When a drowning occurs it is likely to be because throat spasms have prevented breathing or because the person has been immersed in cold water and has developed hypothermia. It is less likely to be because the lungs are full of water – usually only a small amount of water enters the lungs. The water that gushes out of a casualty's mouth is from the stomach and needs to drain away naturally.

Aims of treatment
- restore supply of oxygen to the blood
- arrange removal to hospital

TREATMENT

1 Do not enter the water unless it is absolutely necessary but you need to get the casualty onto dry land.

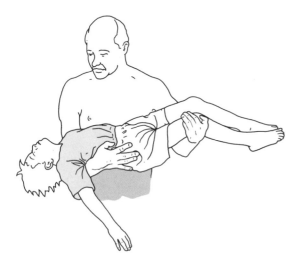

2 If you have to carry the casualty, make sure his head is lower than the rest of his body.
3 Lay the casualty down on coats or blankets, keeping his head low and to one side to allow water to drain.
4 If breathing ceases follow resuscitation sequence and act accordingly. (See pages 2-8).

5 Once the casualty is breathing again, place in the recovery position (see page 8).

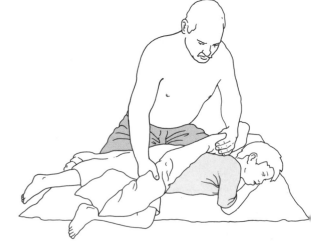

6 To treat hypothermia, remove wet clothing, keep the casualty warm by covering with dry towels or blankets.
7 Make sure the casualty goes to hospital even if apparently recovered.

 DO NOT
- waste time trying to get water out of the casualty's lungs or stomach

SCENARIO

A boy gets into trouble in your swimming lesson.

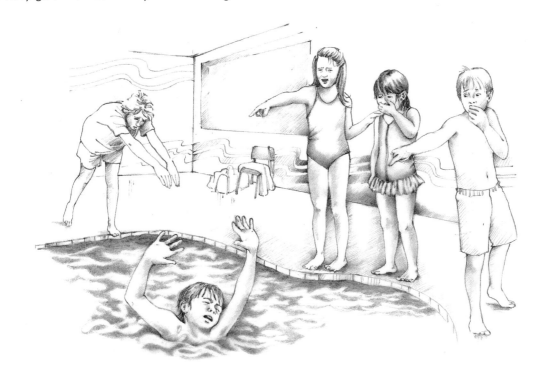

A Should you try to remove water from the boy's lungs?

B Must you always remove the casualty from the water before treating?

Assess

Check the boy is breathing.

Make safe

Lift his head out of the water. Call for help to clear the pool.

Get Help

Dial 999 for an ambulance.

Aftermath

Follow normal procedures for reporting an accident.

Emergency Aid

- Get the boy on to the side.
- Do DRABC assessment and act on findings.
- If normal breathing starts, place casualty on blanket, remove wet clothing, cover with warm, dry blanket or towels, and place in recovery position (see page 8).
- Arrange for casualty to go to hospital even if he recovers quickly.

ESSENTIAL INFORMATION

The nervous system – the brain, spinal cord and nerves – controls all movement and vital body functions, such as breathing and circulation. Anything which upsets the normal functioning of the brain may lead to unconsciousness. An unconscious person, unlike someone who is merely sleeping, may not respond to stimuli such as shouting or pinching. Normal reflexes may fail to work: if a person is lying face up, the tongue may fall back in the throat and block the airway, causing the person to asphyxiate.

Any unconscious casualty requires immediate Emergency Aid.

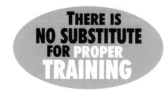

THERE IS NO SUBSTITUTE FOR PROPER TRAINING

Main causes of unconsciousness

Unconsciousness may be due to:

Damage to brain itself	Head injury
Blood not reaching brain	Stroke; heart attack; fainting; shock
Changes in chemical content of blood reaching brain	Hypoglycaemia (low blood sugar); poisoning (including alcohol and drugs)
Other conditions	E.g. epilepsy

People who suffer from diabetes (who are the most likely to have a hypoglycaemia attack) or epilepsy usually carry warning cards or wear bracelets.

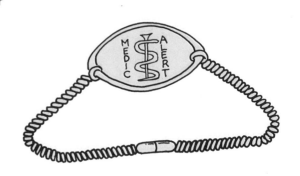

I AM A DIABETIC ON INSULIN

Name_____

Address_____

_____

Telephone_____

If I am found ill, please give me 2 teaspoons of sugar in a small amount of water or 3 of the glucose tablets which I am carrying.
If I fail to recover in 10 minutes, please call an ambulance (Dial 999).
The British Diabetic Association
10 Queen Anne Street, London W1M 0BD

Assessing the level of response

In Emergency Aid an estimate of the casualty's levels of response is important in assessing their condition. A casualty who seems merely drowsy at first, but subsequently loses consciousness, may require special treatment, and recording any changes in level of consciousness can give valuable information to the doctor later.

Eyes	**Movement** - does the casualty	**Speech**
are they open? do they open on command? do they respond to pain? do they remain closed?	respond to commands? move in response to pain? make no response at all?	is it normal? is it confused; inappropriate? is it incomprehensible? does the casualty make no response at all?

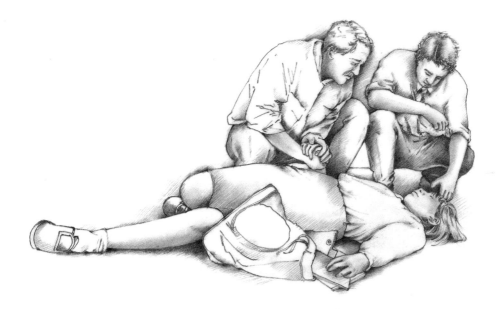

General rules for treating unconsciousness
- Follow the DRABC procedure.
- Assess and record the levels of response.
- Examine the casualty carefully for other injuries.
- Obtain medical aid.

UNCONSCIOUS CASUALTY

Aims of treatment
* keep the airway open
* assess and record levels of response
* treat injuries, if possible
* get proper medical help

TREATMENT

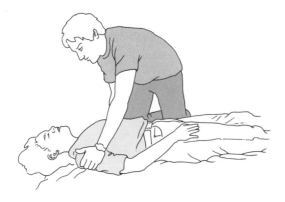 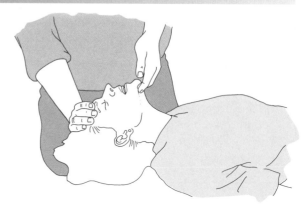

1 Check for and clear any danger.
2 'Shout and shake' – speak loudly and gently shake by the shoulders.
3 If there is no response, open the airway by lifting the chin and tilting the head back.
4 Check breathing.
5 If the casualty is breathing place in the recovery position (see page 8).
6 Check pulse.
7 Check for and control severe bleeding (see page 35).
8 Loosen tight clothing and examine carefully from head to toe for signs of injury. Support suspected fractures (see page 60).

Call an ambulance immediately. Remain with the casualty. Check breathing and pulse frequently. If either stops follow the resuscitation sequence.

Continue to assess and record levels of response every ten minutes.

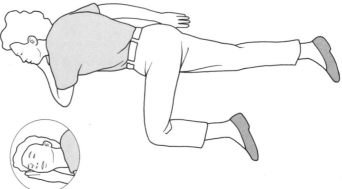

SCENARIO

A pupil collapses during morning assembly.

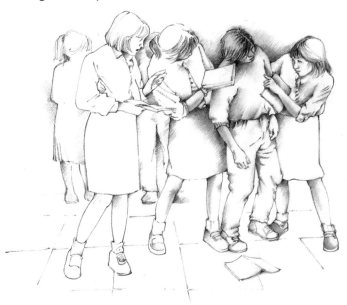

A What procedures would you follow to assess levels of response?

B If the pupil is not fully conscious, what would you do?

Assess

All you know is that a child is unconscious.

- Find out what happened from other pupils. They may have noticed something which will help to diagnose what's wrong.
- Find out urgently if he has a particular condition which may have triggered the collapse.

Make safe

Move other pupils away from the area to avoid crowding or distressing the boy.

Get Help

You will probably have already sent for help.

Aftermath

Carry out the normal reporting procedures.

Emergency Aid

- Check for danger.
- 'Shout and shake'.
- Open airway, check breathing.
- Turn casualty into recovery position (see page 8).
- Check pulse.
- Check for and control severe bleeding.
- Examine carefully for any injuries sustained during fall.
- Stay with him until fully recovered, continuing to monitor and record levels of response.

If no response, follow procedures for unconscious casualty (as opposite).
Dial 999.

HEAD INJURIES AND CONCUSSION

Any head injury is potentially dangerous and demands medical attention, especially if the casualty becomes unconscious. If the pupils of the eyes are uneven in size, this may be a sign of more serious head injuries.

A blow to the head or jaw, or even indirect force from a heavy fall, may also cause *concussion*, in which the brain is 'shaken' within the skull.

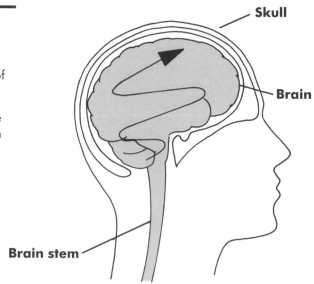

Skull

Brain

Brain stem

Recognition
- brief loss of consciousness
- dizziness; nausea
- short memory loss; headache

Aims of treatment
- monitor casualty until fully recovered
- obtain medical aid, if necessary

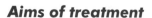

TREATMENT

1 If the injury seems minor and the casualty remains conscious, monitor levels of response (see page 19) for any worsening of her condition.

2 If the casualty loses consciousness, or her condition deteriorates, follow the usual procedures for an unconscious casualty (see page 20).

3 Check for any other signs of injury, e.g. bleeding from scalp, ear or nose; bruising developing in or around eye. These may indicate possible skull fracture.

4 Place in the recovery position (see page 8). Dial 999 for an ambulance. Continue to monitor breathing, pulse and levels of response.

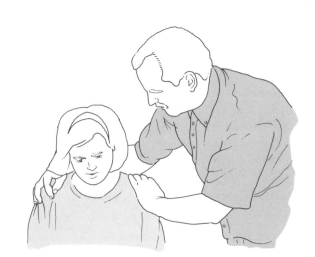

Even after apparent recovery, the casualty should be seen by a doctor as soon as possible. There may be delayed effects or possible internal injury.

SCENARIO

A boy has been accidentally kicked in the head during a rugby match. He seems partially conscious, but dazed and confused.

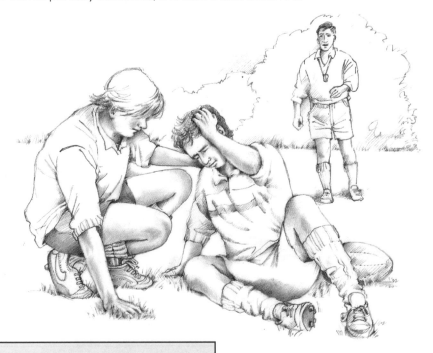

A If his condition deteriorates or he loses consciousness, what should you do first?

B What particular signs of injury should you look for?

Assess

The boy appears to be concussed, but the blow to the head may have caused more serious, but not immediately apparent, injuries.

Make safe

Make sure the boy lies still and ask other team members to stand back and to give you space to work safely.

Get Help

You will have sent for help immediately.

Aftermath

Carry out the normal reporting procedures. Ensure the casualty sees a doctor.

Emergency Aid

- Check breathing and pulse (see page 3).
- Assess levels of response (see page 19).
- Check for other signs of injury.
- If possible, wrap some warm, dry, material (such as a tracksuit) under and over him.
- If breathing deteriorates or he loses consciousness, carry out the initial assessment (see page 2) and place in the recovery position.

HYPOGLYCAEMIA

This occurs when the blood sugar level falls well below normal and causes a chemical change to the brain. It is found most often in people who have *diabetes*, a condition in which the body is unable to regulate the concentration of sugar in the blood. Diabetics control this through insulin injections or tablets. Hypoglycaemia may occur as a result of missed meals, over-exertion, or if too much insulin is taken.

Recognition
- sweating; pale and clammy skin
- shallow breathing
- faintness; confused, disoriented or even aggressive behaviour
- in more severe cases, the person may become unconscious

Aims of treatment
- monitor casualty until fully recovered
- obtain medical aid, if necessary

TREATMENT

1 If he is conscious, help the casualty to sit or lie down and immediately give something sugary.
2 Let him rest until fully recovered. Continue to give sweet food or drink.

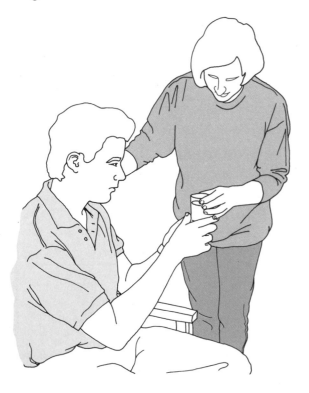

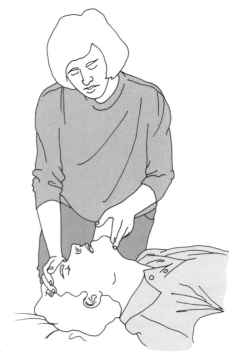

3 If he becomes unconscious, open the airway. Follow the normal procedure for an unconscious casualty (see page 20).
4 Place in the recovery position (see page 8) and call an ambulance immediately.

SCENARIO

Your next class has just had P.E. A girl you know to be diabetic is obviously ill, and is being supported by her friends.

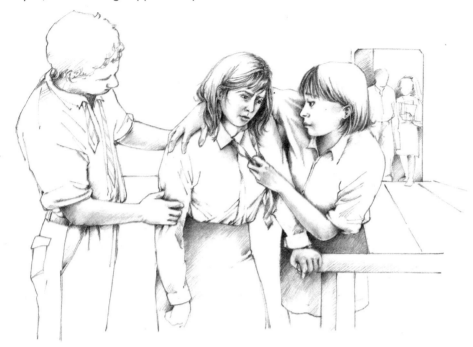

A How could you tell that the girl is having a hypoglycaemia attack?

B What is she likely to be carrying?

Assess

You know that the girl is a diabetic. Her pale, clammy skin and shallow breathing indicate a hypoglycaemia attack.

Make safe

Clear a space around the girl and help her sit or lie down.

Get Help

Obtain medical aid urgently if the casualty is unconscious.

Aftermath

Let the girl's parents know what has happened and encourage them to inform the girl's doctor.

Emergency Aid

- As a diabetic, she may be carrying sugar lumps. Give these to her or any other sweet food or drink which is available.
- Let her rest for a while. Give her more sweet food or drink.
- If she should become unconscious, follow normal procedures for unconsciousness (see page 20), place in the recovery position and call an ambulance.

EPILEPSY

Epilepsy is a condition in which disturbance in the function of the brain may cause fits. Fits are characterised by involuntary contractions of muscles and are usually accompanied by loss of consciousness.

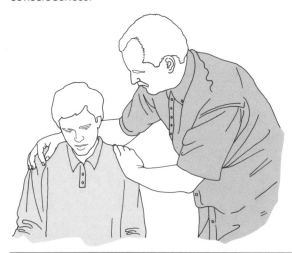

Aims of treatment
* protect from injury during fit
* ensure follow up care, as necessary

Minor epileptic attacks

These may pass unnoticed. Symptoms may include: staring blankly, as though daydreaming; slight twitching of mouth, eyelids or head; unusual behaviour – smacking or chewing lips, fiddling with clothes, making strange noises.
Treatment: Get the person to sit down in a quiet place, away from any possible danger; talk to him calmly, keeping other people away. If he is unaware of the condition, he should see a doctor. Other people should be informed as appropriate.

TREATMENT

Major epileptic attacks

Symptoms may include: sudden unconsciousness, followed by becoming rigid; convulsive jerking movements, often violent; saliva may appear at the mouth; jaw may be clenched; breathing noisy; there may be loss of bladder or bowel control. Then muscles relax and breathing becomes normal. The casualty recovers consciousness, usually within a few minutes. He may feel dazed, though unaware of what has happened.

1 If you see the casualty collapsing, try to ensure he does not injure himself.
2 Ask anyone nearby to move clear.
3 Gently loosen clothing around the neck; if possible cushion his head.
4 When convulsions stop, place in the recovery position (see page 8).
5 If he goes into another fit call an ambulance.
6 Stay with the casualty until he is completely recovered or an ambulance arrives.

▨▨▨ DO NOT ▨▨▨
* try to restrain the person during the fit
* move (unless in physical danger) or attempt to wake him
* try to open mouth and put anything in it

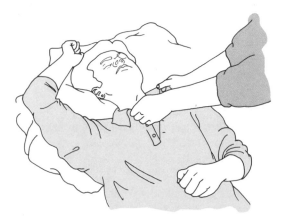

ESSENTIAL INFORMATION

The circulatory system – the heart and blood vessels (arteries, veins and capillaries) – distributes blood to all parts of the body, so that oxygen and nutrients reach the tissues and waste products are carried away.

The circulatory system may fail if:

1 Serious bleeding or a heart disorder reduces the volume of blood circulating, thus causing shock to develop. The tissues – and most importantly the brain – are deprived of oxygen. The priority in Emergency Aid is to act swiftly to improve the blood supply to the brain.

2 The heart stops beating. Immediate action is essential to prevent brain damage and to save the casualty's life. The priority here is to get the blood circulating again by artificial means, i.e. chest compression.

Checking for the heartbeat

Each time the heart beats, a pulse – or wave of pressure – passes through the arteries. This can be felt most easily at the wrist (radial pulse) and neck (carotid pulse) where an artery lies close to the surface of the body. In Emergency Aid it is advisable to check the carotid pulse because even a weak pulse can be felt there.

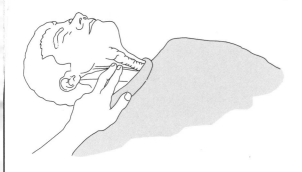

Taking the carotid pulse

1 Locate the carotid pulse in the hollow between the voice box and the main muscle of the neck.
2 Take the pulse by pressing your finger tips gently on the artery.
3 Check for up to ten seconds before deciding that the pulse is absent.
4 If it is present, feel for one minute to check:
   * rate – the pulse rate in a normal adult is between 60 and 80 beats a minute; in a child it is faster
   * strength
   * regularity

The pulse may quicken as a result of exertion, fear, loss of blood. It may slow as a result of fainting and some heart disorders.

General rules for treating circulatory emergencies

* Carry out DRABC procedure: danger, response, airway, breathing, circulation.
* Act immediately to improve blood supply to the brain.
* If the heart stops, get the blood and oxygen circulating again by artificial ventilation and chest compression.
* Obtain medical aid immediately.

SHOCK

Shock will develop if the circulatory system fails and insufficient oxygen reaches the tissues. The body's defence is to try to direct blood to the brain and other vital organs, away from less important areas, such as the skin. The symptoms of shock relate to this redistribution of blood.

Shock may follow many injuries. It can develop in cases where:
- the heart fails to pump blood, e.g. in a heart attack.
- there is heavy loss of bodily fluids, e.g. external or internal bleeding, severe burns, prolonged vomiting or diarrhoea.
- there is extreme pain or fear.

Recognition
- skin colour becomes pale, grey (most clearly seen inside lips); skin feels cold, clammy
- rapid, weak pulse
- rapid, shallow breathing
- casualty may feel faint, nauseous, thirsty

If not enough oxygen reaches the brain, the casualty may become restless, even aggressive; may gasp for air. Finally, she may lose consciousness. In extreme cases, the heart stops.

Aims of treatment
- improve blood supply to vital organs
- treat any injuries e.g. bleeding, burns
- send to hospital urgently

TREATMENT

1 Treat any obvious injuries, such as bleeding or burns (see Chapter 4 or 5).
2 Lay the casualty down (unless injuries put her at risk); reassure constantly, keeping her as still and calm as possible.
3 Raise her legs and loosen any tight clothing.
4 Protect from cold by using coats or blankets.
5 Check breathing, pulse and levels of response (see page 19).

6 If casualty loses consciousness, follow the resuscitation sequence (see page 3); place in recovery position (see page 8).

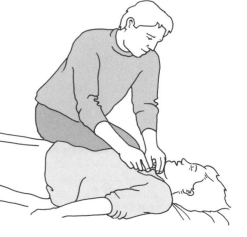

DO NOT
- apply direct heat
- let casualty eat or drink anything
- leave alone at any time
- let the casualty smoke

SCENARIO

A pupil has been knocked down outside the school gates by a car.

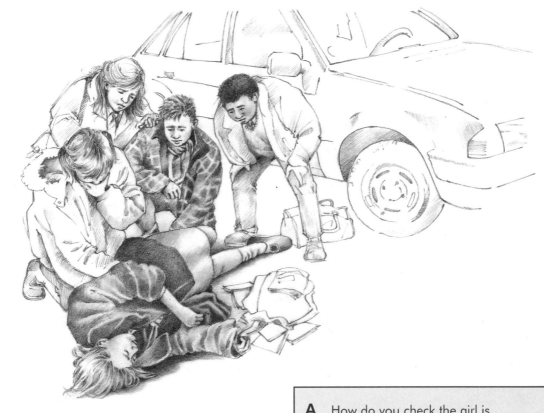

A How do you check the girl is conscious?
B Which pulse should you take?
C How will you keep her warm?

Assess

The girl is conscious; no injuries are immediately apparent. Shock may develop.

Make safe

Clear the area of people and traffic.

Get Help

Dial 999.

Aftermath

Follow normal procedure for informing others.

Emergency Aid _____

- Lay the girl down and check carefully for signs of injury. Place something under her feet to raise her legs.
- Loosen tight clothing.
- Keep her warm, using coats, etc. Put them underneath as well as on top.
- Monitor for breathing and pulse, and for signs of shock.

FAINTING

Fainting is a very short loss of consciousness, normally followed by swift and complete recovery. A faint is caused by a temporary reduction in the flow of blood to the brain, and may be brought on by emotional distress; pain or fear; lack of food or sleep. It more often occurs after someone has been standing still for a long time, especially in a warm or stuffy atmosphere.

A person about to faint will feel weak and giddy, possibly nauseous. Other signs are very pale skin and a slow pulse.

Aim of treatment
- improve blood supply to brain

TREATMENT

1 Lie the casualty down and raise his legs above the level of the heart. Loosen any tight clothing.
2 Make sure he has plenty of air: move any onlookers away; fan air onto his face; open windows, as appropriate.
3 Monitor breathing and pulse.
4 As he recovers help him to sit up gradually.
5 Seek qualified help if you are worried about his condition.

6 If he does not regain consciousness quickly, place him in the recovery position (see page 8) and dial 999 for an ambulance.

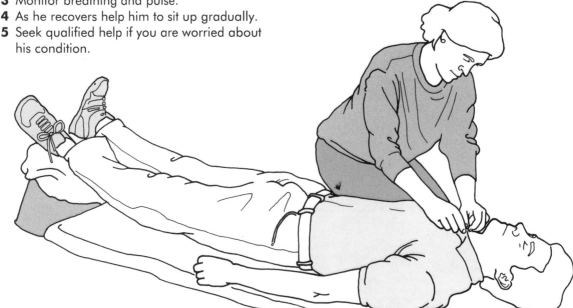

//// DO NOT ////
- give any alcohol
- give anything to drink or eat until fully recovered

HEART DISORDERS

Blood is supplied to the heart by the coronary arteries. If this supply is reduced or obstructed the heart cannot function properly and may stop altogether.

Angina Pectoris

This condition is caused by the narrowing of coronary arteries. An angina attack may be brought on by over-exertion and is most often characterised by severe pain in the chest, a feeling of weakness and breathlessness. A known angina sufferer will almost certainly carry medication.

Aim of treatment
* minimise strain on the heart

TREATMENT

1 Follow DRABC procedure and if the casualty is conscious:
2 Help the casualty to sit down quietly and rest. Attacks normally last only a few minutes.
3 Find out if the casualty has medication to treat the attack.

4 If rest and/or medication do not ease the pain within about three minutes, dial 999 for an ambulance.
5 Monitor response, breathing and pulse and be prepared to resuscitate if necessary (see page 32).

Heart attack

A heart attack is most often caused by a sudden obstruction, such as a clot, in one of the coronary arteries.

Recognition
* crushing pain in the chest (which may feel similar to severe indigestion), which – unlike angina – does not go away with rest
* ashen skin, blue lips; breathlessness
* collapse, often without warning
* rapid pulse, becoming weaker and irregular

Aims of treatment
* minimise the strain on the heart
* transfer to hospital without delay

TREATMENT

1 Follow the DRABC procedure and if the casualty is conscious:
2 Help the casualty into a half-sitting position, supporting knees and shoulders with blankets or jackets. Loosen tight clothing.
3 If one is available, advise him to chew an ordinary aspirin slowly.
4 Get someone to call an ambulance and report a suspected heart attack.
5 Keep checking breathing and pulse.
6 If he loses consciousness follow the resuscitation sequence (see page 3) and place in recovery position (see page 8) - provided he is breathing.

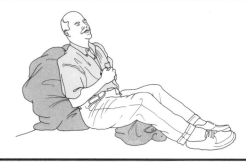

▰▰▰ DO NOT ▰▰▰
* attempt chest compression unless the heart has stopped

CARDIAC ARREST

Cardiac arrest means sudden stopping of the heart. The most common cause is a heart attack; it may also be due to massive electric shock; drug overdose; suffocation; very heavy loss of blood. The casualty loses consciousness; heartbeat and breathing cease.

Prompt action can prevent brain damage and save a person's life. This involves a regular cycle of chest compression with mouth-to-mouth ventilation. It is unlikely that the heart will actually restart before expert assistance is given, but this life-saving cycle will help oxygenated blood reach the heart and the brain.

Aim of treatment

- ensure that oxygen reaches the heart muscle and brain

TREATMENT - ADULT

If during the DRABC assessment you find that the casualty is not breathing:

If you are on your own:
1 Dial 999 for an ambulance immediately.
2 On your return quickly reassess DRAB.
3 If still not breathing give 2 ventilations.
4 Check the pulse.
5 If there is no pulse give 15 chest compressions followed by 2 ventilations.
6 Continue to give 15 compressions to every 2 ventilations until help arrives.
7 Only if the casualty's colour improves check the pulse.
8 If the pulse is present stop chest compressions and continue to ventilate if necessary.

If you have help:
1 One person should go to dial 999 for an ambulance while the other immediately starts CPR (see left).
2 When the helper returns they should treat any other life threatening conditions and be prepared to take over if the person doing CPR tires.

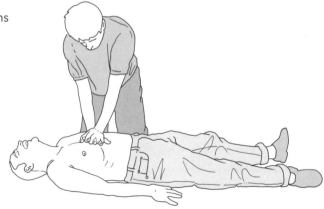

TREATMENT - CHILD

If, while carrying out the DRABC assessment, you find that the casualty is not breathing:

1 Give five breaths of mouth-to-mouth ventilation (see page 6).
2 Check circulation (see page 3).
3 If there is no pulse commence CPR.

If you are on your own:

1 Give 5 chest compressions at the rate of 100 compressions per minute (see page 7).
2 After 5 compressions give <u>one</u> breath of mouth-to-mouth ventilation (see page 6).
3 Continue this process for one minute.
4 If the child is small enough, carry him to the telephone and dial 999 for an ambulance.
5 If you have left the child to dial 999, on your return quickly reassess the DRABC (as above).
6 Continue resuscitation, 5 compressions to one breath until the ambulance arrives.
7 Only if the casualty's colour improves check the pulse.
8 If the pulse is present stop chest compressions and continue to ventilate if necessary.

If you have help:

1 One person should go to dial 999 for an ambulance while the other immediately starts CPR (see left).
2 When the helper returns they should treat any other life threatening conditions and be prepared to take over if the person doing CPR tires.

SCENARIO

An older member of staff collapses suddenly during a staff meeting.

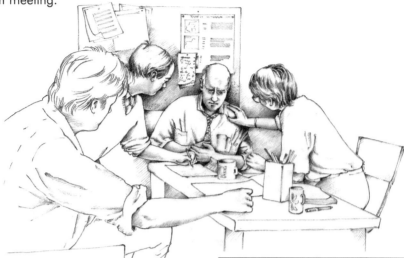

A What should be your first priority?

B What treatment do you give if the casualty has a pulse?

C What do you do if there is no pulse?

Assess

Your colleague has turned very pale and clutches at his chest. Then he loses consciousness. These signs, combined with the suddenness of his collapse, lead you to suspect a heart attack.

Aftermath

Follow normal procedures for informing others.

Emergency Aid

- Get a colleague to dial 999 immediately. While waiting for the ambulance, follow the DRABC procedure:

Airway
- Open the airway.

Breathing
- Check breathing.

If he is not breathing:

- Place him flat on his back.
- Clear any obstruction from the mouth.
- Give two breaths of mouth-to-mouth ventilation (see page 4).
- Check pulse.

If he has a carotid pulse:

- Give mouth-to-mouth ventilation, at a rate of about ten breaths per minute.
- Check for pulse after each minute.

If there is no carotid pulse:

Circulation
- Give 15 chest compressions (see previous page).
- Give two breaths of mouth-to-mouth ventilation.
- Repeat the cycle: 15 compressions to two ventilations – until the ambulance arrives.
- Only if the casualty's colour improves, check the pulse.
- Stop chest compressions if the pulse is present and continue to ventilate if necessary.

ESSENTIAL INFORMATION

Most wounds are characterised by external bleeding, i.e. blood is lost through cut, torn or punctured skin. Severe external bleeding can be dramatic and distressing, both for the casualty and for you. It may lead to shock, and occasionally to unconsciousness.

The first priority in Emergency Aid is to stop (or at least slow down) the bleeding. There are three simple but important techniques involved here:

1 **Direct pressure**, i.e. pressing directly on the wound to flatten surrounding blood vessels and slow blood loss.
2 **Elevation**, i.e. raising the injured area above the heart, to reduce blood flow to the wound.
3 **Lay casualty down**, this may help because it will reduce the flow to the site of the injury, and minimise shock.

First Aid Hygiene, HIV and Hepatitis B

These are both viral infections that can be spread by blood to blood contact. With a little thought and pre-planning the risk of infection can be minimised.

- All blood can be a potential hazard to the first aider so avoid unnecessary unprotected contact.
- Cover any wounds or open sores you may have with a waterproof dressing.
- The use of good quality disposable latex gloves is strongly recommended.
- Good handwashing prior to treating minor wounds will protect the casualty from infection.
- Washing your hands prior to taking off contaminated gloves and again afterwards, will provide you with protection from infection.
- Blood will not pose a problem on your undamaged skin, but to minimise risk, wash off any blood as soon as possible with soap and water. If the eye or mouth or damaged skin is infected, then seek medical advice.
- Dispose of any contaminated dressings etc into yellow clinical waste sacks. These should then be incinerated.

- Clean up blood spills using an appropriate product (eg bleach granules) according to instructions. If not available, then use absorbent paper towels and bleach. After this has been cleared, then the area should be dried and waste matter disposed of in yellow sacks for incineration.

NB: *Care must be taken to ensure adequate ventilation when using the above products. Gloves should be worn when cleaning blood spillage.*

No evidence has been shown that HIV is spread by mouth-to-mouth resuscitation. If you are at all worried, then the use of a simple face shield or mask will provide protection.
The lack of shields, gloves, etc should not deter any first aider from providing assistance at the scene if an accident.
Contaminated needles are a particular risk, so great care must be taken when dealing with them. Disposal must be in a recognised sharps box.

General rules for treating bleeding
- Control the bleeding.
- Reduce risk of infection, both to the casualty and yourself.
- Act to minimise shock.
- Obtain medical aid (unless the wound is superficial).

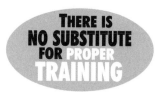

THERE IS
NO SUBSTITUTE
FOR PROPER
TRAINING

SEVERE EXTERNAL BLEEDING

Aims of treatment
- control bleeding
- minimise shock
- reduce any risk of infection
- arrange urgent removal to hospital

TREATMENT

1 Apply direct pressure, preferably over a pad until a dressing is available.
This will help the blood to clot.

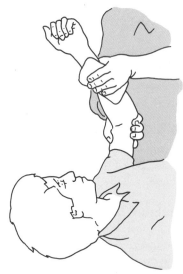

2 Raise and support the injured limb to help slow the bleeding (unless you suspect a fracture).

3 Lay the casualty down to reduce the blood flow to the site of the injury and minimise shock.

⚠ DO NOT ⚠

- remove pads which are soaked with blood – simply place new ones on top
- lose time looking for dressings – the vital Emergency Aid is to stop the bleeding
- apply a tourniquet – it can make bleeding worse and lead to tissue damage

---

4 Place a sterile dressing over the pad. Bandage securely, but not too tightly as this may interfere with normal circulation.

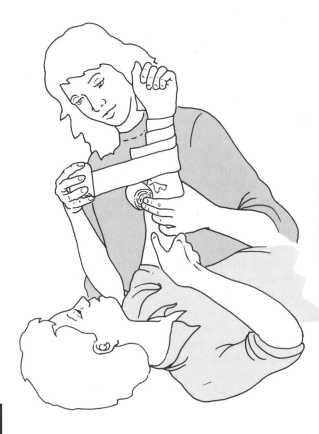

5 If the wound continues to bleed, bandage another dressing over the top.
6 Treat for shock, as necessary (see page 28).
If you can, raise his legs to help reduce shock and slow the flow of blood to the wound.
Loosen tight clothing and protect the casualty from the cold.

SCENARIO

In a Home Economics class a pupil has cut his hand badly with a sharp knife.

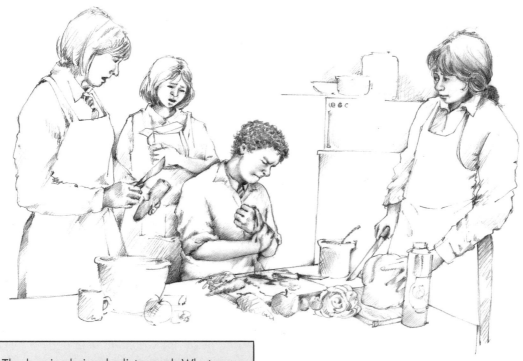

A The boy is obviously distressed. What can you do to minimise shock?

B If there are no First Aid dressings to hand, what do you do?

Assess

There seems to be a lot of blood – but is it as serious as it at first appears? A little blood goes a long way, especially if mixed with water or some other liquid. Nevertheless, you must act without delay.

Make safe

Remove the knife from the floor, in case anyone else gets hurt.

Get Help

You will probably have sent for help.

Aftermath

You should also carry out normal procedures to record an accident.

Emergency Aid

- Apply direct pressure, using a pad if possible (this could be improvised with a clean handkerchief or tissues). Squeeze the edges of the wound together.
- Raise his arm.
- Lie him down and reassure constantly to reduce shock and risk of fainting.
- Maintain the pressure until a dressing is available. Bandage securely.
- Apply a further dressing if blood soaks through.

OBJECT EMBEDDED IN WOUND

If an object, such as a large piece of glass or metal, is embedded in the wound, you must not attempt to pull it out. This would probably make the bleeding worse and could cause tissue damage.

Aims of treatment
• control bleeding without disturbing the object in the wound
• protect from infection

TREATMENT

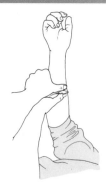 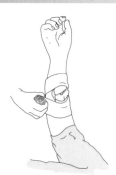

1 Control bleeding by pressing on either side of the embedded object.
2 Raise and support the injured area to help reduce the bleeding.
3 Gently cover the wound and object with a dressing to protect from infection.

4 Taking care not to disturb the dressing or object, build up layers of padding around the wound.
5 Make diagonal turns with a bandage above and below the wound to hold pads in place.
6 Get the casualty to hospital.

MINOR WOUNDS

Wounds which cause minor bleeding are very common in schools. Medical aid is only necessary if the bleeding does not stop or if there is a particular risk of infection.

TREATMENT

1 Wash your hands thoroughly.
2 Clean the wound with running water.
3 Use a clean tissue to pat dry around the area.
4 Cover the wound with an adhesive dressing.

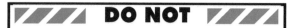 **DO NOT**
• use cotton wool or any other fluffy material to dress the wound

BLEEDING TOOTH SOCKET

This may happen if a tooth is damaged or knocked out as a result of a fall or blow to the jaw; or after a tooth has been extracted.

TREATMENT

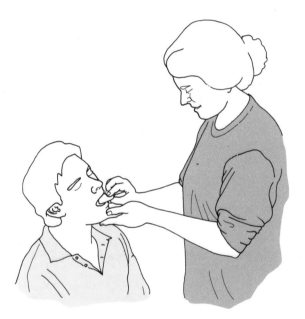

1 Get the casualty to sit down, head forward and tilted towards the injured side. Encourage him not to swallow any blood.
2 Place a pad over the tooth socket. The casualty should bite on this for ten minutes.
3 If bleeding continues, give a clean pad to bite on. If bleeding does not stop after 30 minutes, or it starts again, seek dental or medical help.

> If a tooth is knocked out, try to put it back in the socket, holding it by the crown only (don't touch the root).
> If this is impossible, place the tooth in a cup of milk.
> Get the casualty to a dentist or hospital without delay.

SERIOUS NOSEBLEEDS

Nosebleeds are not usually serious, unless the bleeding is heavy and prolonged. (If they occur after a blow to the head this may indicate a fractured skull, see page 22).

TREATMENT

1 Sit the casualty down and loosen clothing around his neck.
2 Tell him to lean forward and pinch the nostrils together just below the bridge of the nose.
3 He should keep up the pressure for ten minutes, breathing through his mouth all the time. He should avoid swallowing, sniffing or coughing as this may disturb blood clots.
4 If bleeding does not stop after 30 minutes, medical help should be sought.

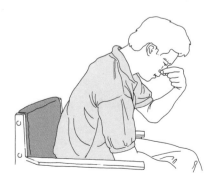

INTERNAL BLEEDING

Internal bleeding may occur if the casualty has been crushed in an accident or had a serious fall. Blood may start to collect within the body's cavities or muscles; later it may leak from an orifice, such as the mouth.

The effects may not be noticeable for some time, but internal bleeding is potentially very dangerous since loss of blood from the circulatory system means loss of oxygen to the brain and other vital organs. Blood collecting within the body can also place pressure on vital organs.

Recognition
- pronounced swelling around the injured area
- severe pain
- rapid, weak pulse
- skin pale, cold and clammy
- bleeding from orifices, such as the mouth or ear
- shock/confusion – possible unconsciousness

Aims of treatment
- minimise shock
- send to hospital urgently

TREATMENT

1 Do not move the casualty unless you have to (e.g. to remove from danger). Do all you can to minimise shock: keep her still and reassure all the time. If possible, raise and support legs. Get someone to call an ambulance.
2 Loosen any tight clothing; keep the casualty warm with blankets or coats.

3 Check and record breathing, pulse and levels of response.
4 If the casualty loses consciousness, carry out resuscitation sequence (see page 3). Place in recovery position (see page 8).
5 Make a note of blood lost from any orifices, and what it looks like – to inform the hospital.

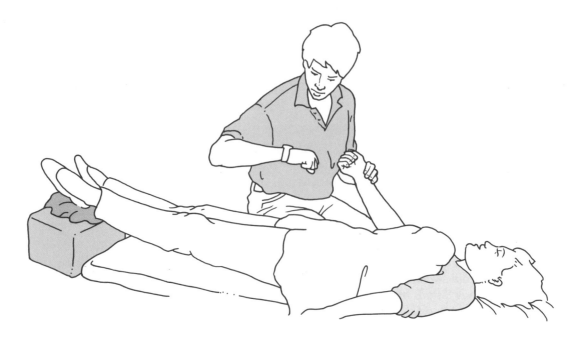

SCENARIO

A pupil has been hit in a road accident. There are no obvious injuries, but he is confused and possibly about to lapse into unconsciousness.

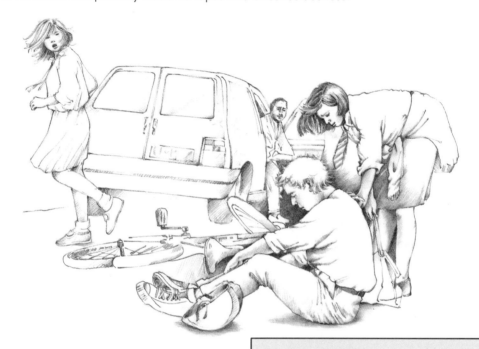

A Would you move the casualty?

B What would you do if the casualty became unconscious?

Assess

There are no obvious injuries, but the severity of the impact/crushing may have caused internal injuries leading to internal bleeding. His confusion and semi-conscious state may be an indication of this.

Look out for other signs: bleeding from the nose, mouth or ear; rapid weak pulse; obvious pain.

Make safe

Make sure there is no further risk of injury to either you or the casualty.

Get Help

You will have sent someone to dial 999 immediately.

Aftermath

Carry out normal reporting procedures.

Emergency Aid

- Check DRABC.
- Do not attempt to move, unless necessary. If possible though, raise and support his legs.
- Cover with warm materials; reassure constantly.
- Assess levels of response (see page 19).
- Monitor breathing and pulse.
- If he does become unconscious, carry out resuscitation sequence (see page 3) and place in recovery position (see page 8).

ESSENTIAL INFORMATION

It is important that you are able to assess the seriousness of burns and scalds, so that you know whether medical aid is required. To make your decision you need to take into account: the cause of the burn or scald; the extent of the burn and its depth.

Causes of burns and scalds

Scalds   wet heat: hot liquids and vapours

Burns   dry burn: flames, hot objects, friction
electrical: low or high voltage current
chemical: industrial chemicals, acids, cleaning fluids, bleaches, etc.
radiation: sunburn
extreme cold: contact with freezing metals or vapours, such as liquid nitrogen

---

Extent of the burn

A burn which covers an extensive area of skin is serious, and will cause shock to develop, whether it is a surface or deep burn.

If a surface burn is smaller than the size of a postage stamp then it may be treated locally. All other burns require medical attention.

Burns involving larger areas of blistering and all full thickness burns will require urgent hospital treatment.

Depth of the burn

Without medical training, it may be difficult to distinguish between surface burns affecting the outer layers of skin and deep burns, though the Emergency Aid is always the same. Some guidelines on what to look for:

- Surface: redness of skin, swelling, tenderness. Can be treated without medical attention (provided the area of the burn is small).
- Partial-thickness: raw skin, blisters. Medical treatment required.
- Full-depth: skin may appear waxy, pale or charred and damage may occur to nerves and muscles beneath skin. Immediate medical attention required.

Airway

This may be affected if toxic smoke, hot gases, corrosive chemicals or extremely hot liquids are involved: tissues swell rapidly, breathing quickly becomes very difficult. Immediate hospital treatment is essential.

General rules for treating burns and scalds
- Make sure of your own safety.
- Stop the burning by means of rapid cooling.
- Cover the affected area.
- Obtain medical aid (unless superficial).

SUPERFICIAL BURNS AND SCALDS

Aims of treatment
- stop the burning
- relieve pain and swelling
- minimise risk of infection

TREATMENT

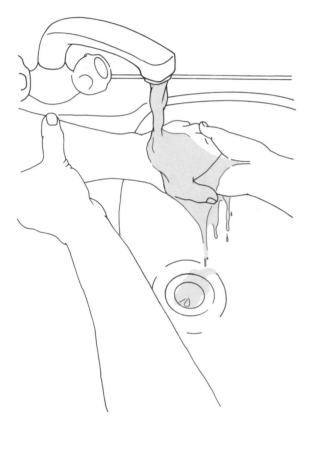

3 To prevent infection, cover the area with a sterile dressing – or any clean, non-fluffy material (e.g. plastic bag, kitchen film, freshly laundered pillow case).

4 Make sure the person is comfortable and reassure if upset.

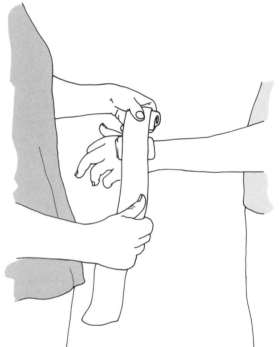

1 Hold the affected area under cold water (or any cold harmless liquid) for at least ten minutes – to stop burning and relieve pain.

2 The injury will probably swell, so you should remove any constricting jewellery, watches or clothing.

DO NOT
- use adhesive dressings
- break blisters
- apply lotions, ointments, creams

SCENARIO
In the science lab, a pupil has knocked over a container of hot liquid. It has spilt onto her arm, and onto the bench.

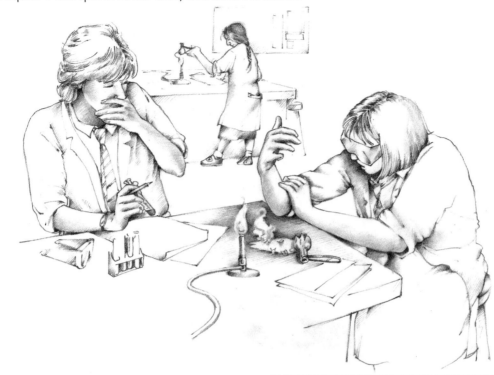

A What is your first priority?
B This is a scald rather than a burn: what should you use to cover it?

Assess
It is obvious that the pupil has been scalded, but you should determine what the liquid is before treating.

Make safe
The Bunsen burner must be turned off. Remove the pupil from the danger area. Ask other class members to stay clear. After treating the pupil, clear debris carefully.

Get Help
Call for medical help if you have not already done so.

Aftermath
Carry out the normal procedure for reporting an accident.

Emergency Aid
- If the scald is from boiling water, pour cold water over the affected area for at least ten minutes. For chemical burns, see page 48.
- Remove any soaked clothing – hot liquid in clothing will make the scald worse and slow the cooling effects of the water.
- Remove anything which may become tight as swelling occurs.
- Cover the area with a clean non-fluffy material.

SEVERE BURNS AND SCALDS

Aims of treatment
- stop the burning and relieve pain
- resuscitate if necessary
- try to prevent infection
- arrange urgent removal to hospital

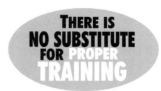

THERE IS
NO SUBSTITUTE
FOR PROPER
TRAINING

TREATMENT

1 Follow the DRABC procedure and start cooling the burn immediately.

2 Make the casualty as comfortable as possible, preferably lying down. Keep talking to calm and reassure him. Get someone to call an ambulance immediately.

3 Continue to pour copious amounts of cold liquid over the burn for at least ten minutes or until the pain is relieved. Remember this may lower the general body temperature as well, so take care to avoid hypothermia.

4 Remove jewellery, watch or clothing from the affected area – unless it is sticking to the skin.

5 Cover the burn with clean non-fluffy material to protect from infection. Cloth, a clean plastic bag or kitchen film all make good dressings.

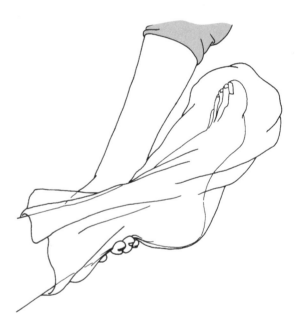

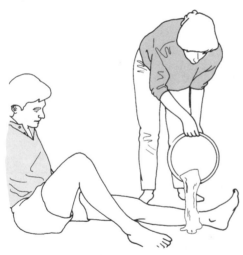

▰▰▰ DO NOT ▰▰▰
- touch injured area
- burst blisters
- apply lotions, ointments, creams
- remove anything which is sticking to the burn

6 Treat for shock while waiting for the ambulance (see page 28). Monitor breathing and pulse.

> If the casualty becomes unconscious, follow the resuscitation sequence, as necessary (see page 3).

SCENARIO

There is a fire in the metalwork workshop.
A pupil's clothing has caught fire.

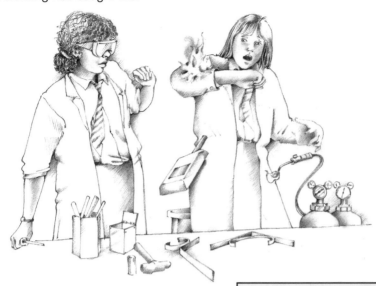

Assess

Follow STOP, DROP and ROLL procedure
* STOP her panicking or running around; any movement or breeze will fan the flames.
* DROP her to the ground.
* If possible WRAP her tightly in a coat, blanket or heavy fabric to smother the flames (DO NOT use nylon, flammable materials or cellular blankets).
* ROLL her along the ground until the flames have been smothered.

Make safe

Make sure the cause of the fire has been removed or turned off.

Get Help

You will have already sent for the ambulance.

Aftermath

Carry out the normal procedure for reporting an accident.

A If there is no water or fire fighting equipment immediately available, what would you do to extinguish the flames?

B What would you do to relieve the pain?

Emergency Aid
* Pour cold water over the burned area for at least ten minutes.
* Remove any watches, rings, belts or tight clothing before any swelling occurs.
* Cover the burn with clean non-fluffy material.
* Treat for shock (see page 28).

CHEMICAL BURNS

Chemical burns develop more slowly than heat burns. Recognition is by:
- intense, stinging pain
- at first, possibly little to see; then redness or staining, blistering and peeling

Aims of treatment
- identify and remove chemical
- minimise burn by cooling
- send casualty to hospital

TREATMENT

1 Follow the DRABC procedure and take precautions to avoid contaminating yourself.

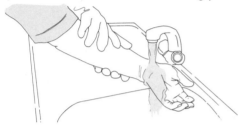

2 Flood the affected area with cold water to prevent further damage to the burned tissue. It will take longer than for a heat burn, so be prepared to do this for 20 minutes. (Try to use slowly running water and make sure that it drains away safely from undamaged areas of skin, as it will be contaminated.)

> If the casualty becomes unconscious, follow the DRABC procedure, as necessary (see page 3).

3 Carefully remove any contaminated clothing. Make sure you do not become a casualty – avoid getting the chemical on your own skin.

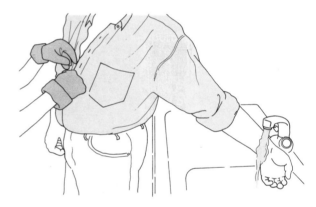

4 Cover the burn with clean, non-fluffy material to protect from infection.
5 Make the casualty comfortable and reassure them. Treat for shock as necessary (see page 28).
6 Get the casualty to hospital without delay.

Chemical burns to the eye

Treat as for other chemical burns, BUT:
- Use cold, gently running water for at least ten minutes to wash away the substance.
- The water must drain off the face without contaminating the uninjured eye.
- Check that both surfaces of the eyelids have been washed. (You may need to pull the eyelids open – be firm but gentle.)
- Cover the eye with clean, non-fluffy material.
- DO NOT let the casualty rub the eye.

It is essential the casualty goes to hospital.

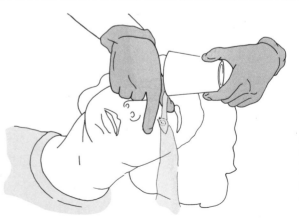

SCENARIO
A pupil spills an unidentified chemical in a Technology lesson.

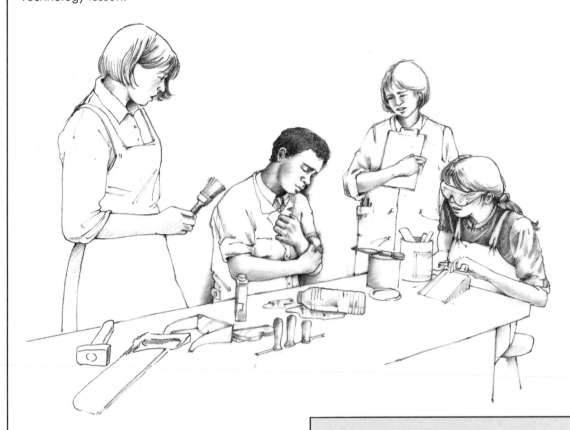

A What signs would tell you that this a chemical burn?

B How do you avoid becoming a casualty yourself?

Assess
Take note of what the casualty says about the cause of the accident and the type of pain. Look for signs of a chemical burn.

Make safe
Make sure that no-one else is in danger and that the source of the burn has been safely removed. Avoid getting the chemical on your own skin.

Get Help
You will have already arranged to get the boy to hospital.

Aftermath
Carry out the normal procedure for reporting an accident.

Emergency Aid
- Flood the affected area with cold water for 20 minutes.
- Remove any contaminated clothing.
- Cover the area with clean, non-fluffy material.
- Make the casualty comfortable; treat for shock (see page 28).

ELECTRICAL BURNS

Visible damage may be seen at the entry and
exit points of the current.
The casualty may be unconscious, with severe
burns (swelling, scorching, charring) and show
signs of shock (see page 28).

TREATMENT

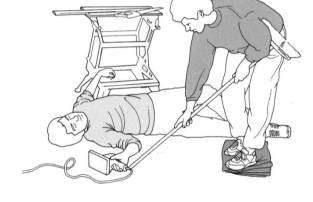

1 Make safe: turn off the electricity if possible;
   make sure the person is no longer in contact
   with the electrical current before you attempt
   to treat him.
2 If you are unable to turn off the current stand
   on dry insulating material such as a rubber or
   plastic mat, or thick pile of newspapers. Use a
   broom, wooden chair or stool to push the
   casualty's limbs away from the source.
3 If the casualty is unconscious,follow the
   DRABC procedure (see page 3). Resuscitate if
   necessary (see page 4). Get someone to call
   an ambulance immediately.
4 Flood the injury with cold water.
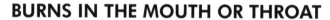
5 Cover the burn with clean, non-fluffy material.
6 Treat for shock (see page 28).

BURNS IN THE MOUTH OR THROAT

A scald from drinking very hot liquid or the
effects of breathing very hot air (for example,
when escaping a fire) can be serious.
The inside of the throat can swell and block the
airway, thus stopping the person from breathing.
The casualty will also be in great pain.

TREATMENT

1 Follow the DRABC procedure. Call medical
   help immediately. Loosen any tight clothing
   around the neck.
2 If the casualty is conscious, give sips of cold
   water at frequent intervals.
3 Keep checking his ABC while waiting for
   medical help to arrive.

4 If the casualty becomes unconscious, place
   in the recovery position. (see page 8)
5 Be prepared to resusitate if necessary.
   (see page 4)

ESSENTIAL INFORMATION

Poisoning occurs when a harmful or toxic substance is taken in sufficient quantity to cause permanent or temporary damage to the body. Poisons may enter the body by:

- inhalation, e.g. toxic gases or fumes; solvents; cannabis etc.
- swallowing, e.g. alcohol; drugs such as painkillers, depressants and stimulants.
- injection, e.g. hypodermic syringe; animal or insect bites or stings.
- absorption through the skin, e.g. household/ garden chemicals, such as paint stripper and certain pesticides.

Once in the body, poisons may work their way into the bloodstream and be carried to the tissues and vital organs.

The Emergency Aid is essentially the same whatever substance is involved, the main differences in treatment depending on whether the casualty is unconscious or conscious, and whether they have burns to the mouth. In addition, you can help to minimise any short or long-term damage by:

1 Trying to find out what the poison is and how much has been taken:
- Check for any signs around the casualty, e.g. a container; smell of fumes.
- Ask the casualty or any bystander what was taken. (Ask the casualty immediately as he may lapse into unconsciousness.)
- Check the casualty for any signs, e.g. alcohol or 'chemical' solvent smell on the breath; blistering or burning on the lips or skin from corrosive chemicals.
- Look at the labels on any containers.

2 When telephoning for medical help, tell the doctor or hospital what you think the casualty has taken: they may be able to give specific advice on what to do while waiting for help to arrive.
3 If the casualty is sick, send a sample of the vomit with them to hospital.

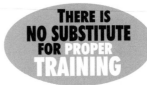

THERE IS NO SUBSTITUTE FOR PROPER TRAINING

General rules for treating poisoning
- Find out all you can about what has been taken and how much.
- Make sure the airway is open and clear, whether the casualty is conscious or unconscious.
- If the casualty is conscious and has burns around the mouth and lips, give sips of water or milk.
- Obtain medical aid.
- Send any suspect containers, tablets, etc. to the hospital/doctor to assist diagnosis.

UNCONSCIOUS CASUALTY

Aims of treatment
- keep the airway open
- assess and record levels of response
- treat injuries, if possible
- get proper medical help
- identify poison, if possible

TREATMENT

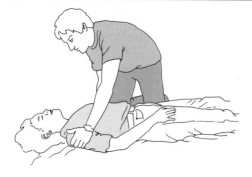

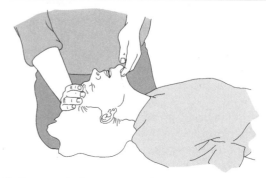

1 Check for and clear any danger.
2 'Shout and shake' – speak loudly and gently shake by the shoulders.
3 If there is no response, check the open the airway: lift the chin and tilt the head back.
4 Check breathing.
5 If the casualty is breathing place in the recovery position (see page 8).
6 Check circulation (pulse and bleeding).
7 Assess and record levels of response (see page 19).
8 Loosen tight clothing and examine carefully from head to toe for signs of injury. Control any bleeding (see page 35); support suspected fractures (see page 60).

Call an ambulance immediately. Remain with the casualty. Check breathing and pulse frequently. If either stops follow the resuscitation sequence.

Continue to assess and record levels of response every ten minutes.

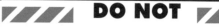

DO NOT

- leave the casualty alone: they may vomit or stop breathing

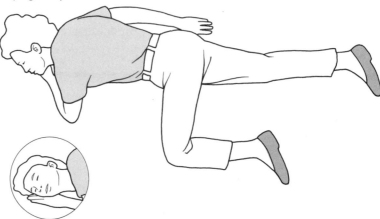

SCENARIO

One evening on a residential trip you discover a group of pupils who have been drinking. One of the group passes out and seems quite deeply unconscious.

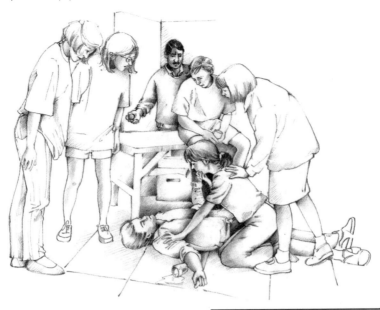

A   What information should you try to find out from other pupils/teachers in your party?

B   What procedures would you follow to assess levels of response?

Assess

- Ask the other pupils exactly what he has been drinking and how much.
- Find out, if you can, if he has a medical condition which may have put him at greater risk. He may be carrying a warning card or bracelet, or one of his friends/another teacher may know.

Make safe

Ensure no other pupil is affected. Remove any remaining alcohol.

Get Help

You will have sent for help immediately. Use your judgement to call either a doctor or an ambulance.

Aftermath

Carry out the normal reporting procedures for when you are away from school.

Emergency Aid

- Check for danger.
- 'Shout and shake'.
- If no response, follow resuscitation sequence (see page 3). Make sure airway is clear.
- If he is breathing normally, place in recovery position (see page 8).
- If he is not breathing, carry out mouth-to-mouth ventilation (see page 4).
- Dial 999 if the casualty is totally unresponsive or fitting.

CONSCIOUS CASUALTY

Aims of treatment

- maintain airway, breathing and circulation
- identify poison, if possible
- obtain medical help

TREATMENT

1 Ask the casualty what happened – she may lose consciousness.

2 If the casualty seems very drowsy or about to pass out, place her in the recovery position (see page 8) to minimise any possible risk of choking on vomit.

3 Keep her warm and calm. Monitor any changes in her condition; assess levels of response (see page 19). Check breathing and pulse every 10 minutes.

4 Send the casualty to hospital. Collect any suspect containers, tablets, powders to send with her.

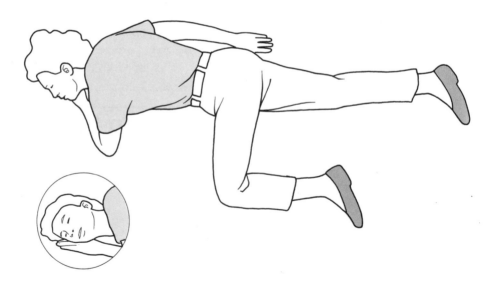

DO NOT

- attempt to make the casualty vomit – it may cause further damage

SCENARIO

After lunch break, a pupil in your class seems intoxicated, but does not appear to have been drinking alcohol; she complains of feeling unwell and having blurred vision.

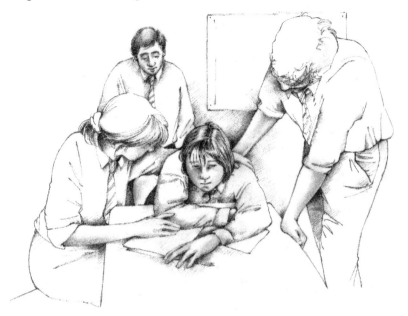

A   What might her symptoms first suggest she has taken?

B   The girl is conscious: why might it be advisable to place her in the recovery position?

Assess

- Ask the girl and other pupils what happened, and what it is she may have taken.
- Does she suffer from diabetes or epilepsy?
- Check her breath/clothes for tell-tale alcohol or 'chemical' solvent smell. Check for any other signs, such as suspect container, plastic bag, syringe, etc.

Make safe

Remove any drugs, solvents or suspect item and keep somewhere safe to send to the hospital/doctor later, if necessary.

Get Help

Send for medical help.

Aftermath

Carry out the normal reporting procedures.

Emergency Aid

- Monitor closely in case she becomes unconscious; assess levels of response.
- Keep her warm and calm. If she becomes distressed, her condition may worsen.
- If her condition does worsen, place her in the recovery position (see page 8) to ensure the airway is kept open.
- Send for medical help.

SPECIFIC DRUG POISONING

Drug poisoning may be caused by misuse of drugs, whether prescribed or illegal – or indeed legal drugs such as alcohol. The risk of poisoning is increased if drugs are mixed (e.g. solvents and alcohol) or if the user has a specific medical condition, e.g. diabetes, epilepsy or heart problems.

A brief summary follows of the main effects of misuse of specific drug types. This may help you both in giving Emergency Aid and in passing on essential information to the hospital. (To obtain more information on drug misuse, see the list of useful addresses on page 71.)

SOLVENTS

glue; aerosol sprays; lighter fuel; etc.
- headaches, nausea, vomiting
- hallucinations
- occasionally unconsciousness, and on rare occasions, heart failure

DEPRESSANTS

barbiturates; tranquillisers
(overdose more likely if taken with alcohol or other drug)
- drowsiness, leading to unconsciousness
- shallow breathing
- weak, irregular pulse or unusually slow or fast pulse

PAINKILLERS

aspirin; paracetamol
- pain, tenderness in upper abdomen
- nausea, vomiting
- unconsciousness, especially if mixed with alcohol or other drug

STIMULANTS AND HALLUCINOGENS

amphetamines; LSD; Ecstasy; cocaine and crack
- excitable, wild behaviour; hyperactivity
- hallucinations
- anxiety; confusion
- sweating; shakiness
- nausea and vomiting

NARCOTICS

heroin; morphine
- pin-point pupils
- shallow breathing; drowsiness, possibly leading to unconsciousness
- nausea, vomiting
- infections from sharing needles

HOUSEHOLD/CHEMICAL

Corrosive chemicals, such as those contained in bleach, paint stripper, weedkiller, etc. can be swallowed, or spilled onto skin, causing chemical burns (see page 48). Normal safety guidelines in schools should mean that such substances are stored under safe conditions. Nevertheless, accidents do happen, and it is important to know the basic Emergency Aid procedures to follow.

Recognition
- swallowed chemicals can burn the lips, mouth and gullet; the mouth may be blistered and/or stained by the chemical burning
- the casualty may vomit

TREATMENT

Follow the usual treatment procedures, depending on whether the casualty is conscious or unconscious. In addition:

- Protect yourself:
  – make sure that there is no spilt chemical or open container which could injure you.
  – if you need to give mouth-to-mouth ventilation, either wash off chemical residue around the casualty's mouth, or cover the mouth with a plastic face shield.

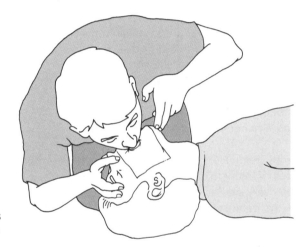

- If the casualty is conscious and there are burns around the lips or mouth, give sips of water or milk.

▰▰▰ **DO NOT** ▰▰▰

- encourage the casualty to vomit as this may intensify the burning

---

Chemical burns
Chemical burns to the eye } see page 48

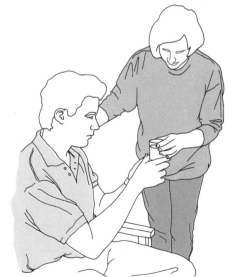

ESSENTIAL INFORMATION

Injuries to bones and muscles – such as fractures and sprains – are fairly common in schools. Unless complicated by further injuries they are not life-threatening, though the wrong action or delayed action may worsen the condition and delay recovery.

The priority in Emergency Aid (particularly with fractures) is therefore to prevent further damage to the bone, muscle or ligament (or to nerves and blood vessels) by avoiding unnecessary movement.

Do not try to do too much: your main aim should be to keep the person still and support the injured part until he or she can see a doctor. Where a fracture is suspected, the casualty should be treated in the position in which you find her – unless she is in immediate danger – before being transferred to hospital.

It may be difficult to distinguish between different types of injury, as the signs and symptoms are often very similar. If in any doubt, you should always treat as for a fracture.

Injuries to bones, muscles and ligaments

Injury	Likely cause
FRACTURE Broken or cracked bone	Direct force, e.g. the impact of something heavy on a bone; or indirect force, e.g. a bad fall
DISLOCATION Bone displaced at a joint	Awkward fall or wrenching force
SPRAIN Tearing or over-stretching of a ligament at or near a joint	Wrenching, twisting movement, e.g. awkward fall
STRAIN Tearing or over-stretching of a muscle ('pulled' muscle)	Awkward movement or violent contraction of muscle (common sporting injury)

General rules for treating bone and muscle injuries
- Avoid moving the casualty, unless at risk of further injury.
- Steady and support the injured part.
- If in doubt about the type of injury, always treat as for a fracture.
- Obtain medical aid.

FRACTURES

There are basic principles which should be followed in treating most fractures. It is, however, important to distinguish between the treatment for closed fractures (below) where there is no open wound around the break, and open fractures (see page 62).

Shock may develop, especially if a major bone is broken or there are associated injuries. A fracture may be complicated by injuries to adjoining muscles or to vital organs.

Recognition
* severe pain, especially on moving
* swelling and bruising
* injured part may look unnatural/out of place
* difficulty in moving the injured part

Aims of treatment
* prevent movement at or near fracture site
* immobilise injured bone to allow safe removal to hospital

TREATMENT

1 Do not move the casualty unless he is in danger of further injury. Keep him still and reassure constantly. Get someone to call an ambulance.

2 Support the limb, but do not move any more than is absolutely necessary.

3 If there is a delay in getting the casualty to hospital, secure the injured part to the trunk or other leg, as appropriate, using padding and bandages or slings.

4 Treat for shock, as necessary (see page 28).

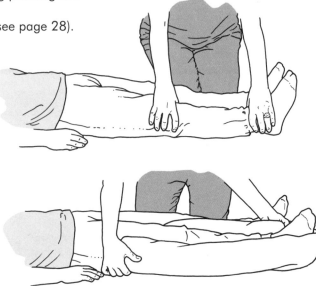

SCENARIO

A pupil has had a fall from her bike in the entrance to the school grounds and has landed heavily and awkwardly on her forearm/wrist.

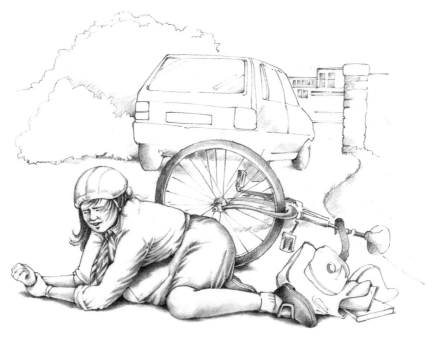

A There may be vehicles entering and leaving the school grounds. Should you move the girl to a safer place?

B What would you do to support and immobilise the injured part?

Assess

The girl complains of sharp pain in her wrist and has virtually no movement there. These symptoms and rapid swelling lead you to suspect a fractured wrist.

Make safe

Remove the bike from the school entrance. Ask a pupil to direct others away from the scene.

Get Help

The casualty must go to hospital.

Aftermath

Carry out normal reporting procedures.

Emergency Aid

- Do not move the girl. Keep her still and reassure constantly to reduce shock. Keep her warm.
- Support the forearm across her chest.
- If possible, surround the forearm with soft padding.
- If you have to wait for help to arrive, ask the girl to support the arm herself while you apply an arm sling, improvised if necessary (see page 65).

OPEN FRACTURES

Open fractures occur when the broken bone pierces the surface of the skin, and the bone is exposed to contamination from the skin and the air. Such fractures require very careful handling to avoid the risk of infection entering the wound or bone.

Aims of treatment
- prevent infection and blood loss.
- prevent movement at or near fracture site
- immobilise injured bone to allow safe removal to hospital

TREATMENT

Cover any wound which exposes a bone with a sterile dressing. Carefully apply direct pressure to slow blood loss (see page 36).

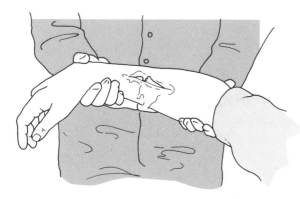

If the bone is sticking out of the wound:
1 On your own, or with help if possible, support the injured part above and below the fracture site and control any bleeding.
2 Gently cover the wound with a dressing to protect from infection.
3 Build up layers of padding around the wound and secure with a bandage, but do not impede the circulation.

Continue treating as for a closed fracture.

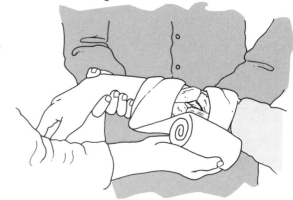

DISLOCATION

The most common sites of dislocation are the shoulder, jaw, thumb and finger.

Treatment
1 Move the injured part as little as possible; at the same time making the casualty as comfortable as you can.
2 Support the injured part with rolled blankets, jacket or cushions, and/or an arm sling.
3 Send for medical help.

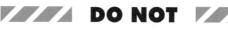 **DO NOT**
- try to replace the bone in its socket

SPRAINS AND STRAINS

Recognition
- pain, especially on moving, or putting weight on a limb
- rapid swelling
- difficulty in moving injured part

REMEMBER: symptoms may be very similar to those of a fracture; if in doubt treat as for a fracture.

Aim of treatment
- reduce pain and swelling

TREATMENT

Follow the **RICE** procedure

R	=	**R**est
I	=	**I**ce
C	=	**C**ompression
E	=	**E**levate

1 Rest and support the injured part so that the casualty is as comfortable as possible.
2 Apply an **Ice** pack to ease pain and reduce swelling. (A Pack of frozen vegetables makes a good ice pack).
3 Compress the injury with a thick layer of padding, firmly secured with a bandage.
4 Elevate the limb to slow blood flow to the injury and thus reduce swelling and bruising.
5 Make sure the casualty sees a doctor, unless the injury seems very minor.

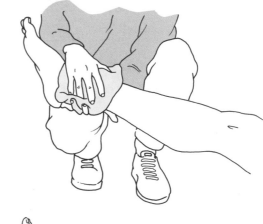

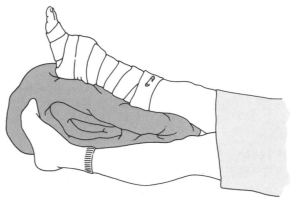

SCENARIO

In the gym a boy has slipped and badly wrenched his ankle.

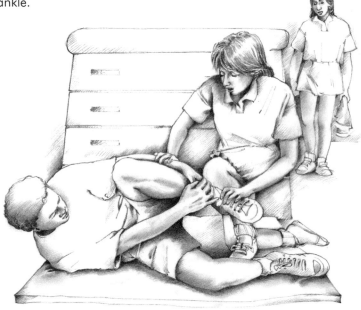

A   What does the mnemonic RICE stand for?

B   What can you do if there is no ice pack available?

Assess

The ankle looks swollen and puffy, and the boy says it feels very painful when he tries to stand. You think it likely he has sprained rather than fractured his ankle.

Make safe

Ask other pupils to leave any apparatus and sit down on the floor while you deal with the boy's injury.

Get Help

You will need an ice pack or water soaked cloth. Obtain medical attention if pain persists or you suspect a fracture.

Aftermath

Carry out normal reporting procedures.

Emergency Aid

- Get the boy to sit or lie still.
- Rest and support the ankle.
- Apply an ice pack or cloth soaked in very cold water.
- Compress the sprain with thick padding, securely bandaged.
- Elevate the ankle.

Encourage the pupil to rest the ankle and see a doctor if the pain and/or swelling does not go away.

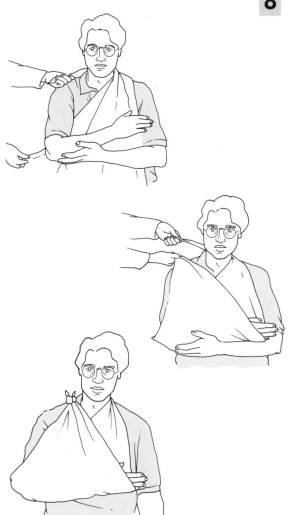

ARM SLINGS

Arm slings are used to support an injured arm or wrist, or dislocated shoulder. They can be made from triangular bandages or strong cloth folded into a triangle.

How to apply

1 Ask the casualty to support the arm if he can. Place bandage between the casualty's arm and chest; take the top end up around the back of the neck.
2 Bring the lower end of the bandage up over the forearm.
3 Tie the two ends together with a reef knot.
4 Bring the point forward and secure it above the elbow with a safety pin.

Emergency arm slings

- If the casualty is wearing a jacket or coat, support the injured arm inside the fastening.

- If the casualty is wearing a jacket, turn the hem up and over the injured arm and pin it securely to the jacket breast.

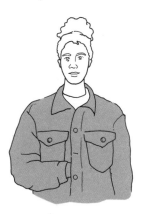

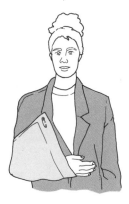

ELEVATION SLINGS

Elevation slings are used to support the arm in cases of collar bone or shoulder injuries; also for hand injuries to control bleeding. Like arm slings, they can be made from triangular bandages or strong cloth folded into a triangle.

How to apply

1 Support the injured side, placing the forearm across the chest so that the fingertips touch the opposite shoulder.
2 Position the bandage over the injured arm with the top end over the shoulder and the point well beyond the elbow.
3 Tuck the base of the bandage under her forearm and elbow.
4 Take the lower end up around her back to meet the top end. Secure with a reef knot just above the collar bone.
5 Tuck in the point of the bandage and secure it above the elbow with a safety pin.

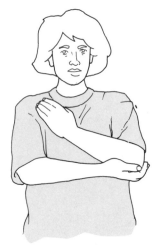

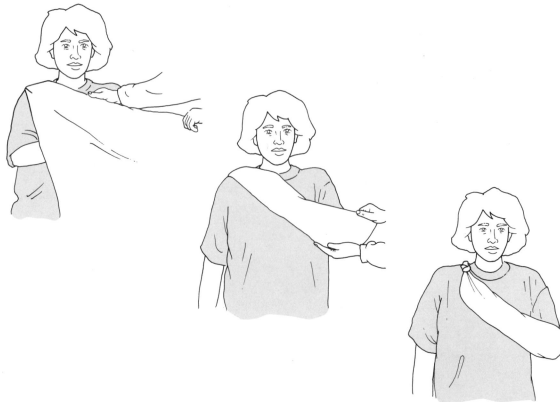

FURTHER TRAINING

This book has provided you with the guidance that you need to give Emergency Aid. It is, however, no real substitute for a proper First Aid course. Mouth-to-mouth Ventilation (page 4) and Chest Compression (page 5) must be practised under qualified supervision and this is why you are reminded throughout the text that there is:

No substitute for proper training

Many Local Education authorities already organise First Aid courses in partnership with St. John Ambulance and it is worth enquiring whether one is available in your locality. Typically, a group of teachers get together and ask for a course and receive training at their school from St. John Ambulance Trainers.

Please, then, consider taking a St. John course. The following are offered in all Counties in England and Wales.

Emergency Aid in Schools course
(6 hours instruction)
This is practical training on most of the topics covered by this book.

Essentials of First Aid course
(16 hours instruction)
This is a longer course for young people, designed to train them to deal with a wide range of First Aid situations.

First Aid at Work course
(24 hours instruction)
This is a course which leads to the statutory certificate recognised by the Health and Safety Executive. It is additionally a useful extra qualification for *school leavers* as it is valued by employers who, by law, have to provide qualified First Aiders on their premises.

Emergency Aid courses
(4 hours instruction)
These are short introductory courses containing a wide range of information. They can be modified to meet the needs of the general public or the Appointed Person in the work place.

Lifesaver First Aid courses
St. John Ambulance has introduced a new range of courses which involve the student more in the learning process. The courses form a programme and you can decide which parts of the programme are relevant to you. These courses are designed to enable you to be confident and competent in the skills at the end of the course.

The courses include:

Lifesaver First Aid course (8 hours)
This course covers the basic lifesaving techniques for an adult.

Lifesaver Plus Course
(16 hours + 2 hours optional examination)
This course assumes knowledge of the Lifesaver course and builds on it by adding information on a wide range of injuries and conditions.

Lifesaver for Babies and Children
(4 hours)
This course stands alone and deals with the lifesaving techniques for babies and children.

Other courses will become available on specialist topics. (e.g. Fractures)

Details of all St. John courses are available in your County. (See the list of addresses on page 70.)
The address of St. John Ambulance Headquarters is:
1 Grosvenor Crescent
London SW1X 7EF
Tel: 0171 235 5231 Fax: 0171 235 0796

TEACHING CHILDREN FIRST AID

The Three Cross Award

The Three Cross Award is suitable for primary and secondary pupils from the age of nine. It also provides useful basic Emergency Aid training for youth groups, and is used and recognised in a wide variety of voluntary and statutory youth organisations. The success of the scheme is evidenced by the thousands of certificates that are issued every year.

The awards are progressive, with the One Cross awarded at primary level and the Two and Three Cross at secondary level, (depending on the ability of the group). Participants practise their Emergency Aid skills and are awarded badges and certificates as their proficiency increases and they demonstrate competency in each skill.

Resource Materials
The core of the three-part training programme is a 42 minute video, which can be shown over a series of training sessions. Emergency Aid techniques are discussed and explained, and then demonstrated by young people. The video is based on the three levels - One, Two and Three Cross.

Included with the video is a booklet providing guidance on teaching objectives and advice on assessment. St. John Ambulance also supplies competitively priced First Aid text books and manuals to accompany the video and a 'Student Refresher Booklet' for participants who have completed the course.

The badges, certificates, video and all other resource materials are available from:
St. John Supplies,
PO Box 707B, Friend Street,
London, EC1V 7NE.
Tel:0171 278 7888 Fax: 0171 837 1642

Uses
Within school the Three Cross Award is very flexible, and can fit a range of curriculum activities, either on its own or with additional First Aid elements. The most popular applications are:

- Local Junior Citizenship schemes
- PSE, PSHE, and PE lessons
- General National Vocational Qualifications
- City & Guilds Certificates
- Junior Sports Leader & Community Sports Leader awards
- Outside school, the Scout and Guide Associations (amongst others) recognise the Award for their badge schemes.

For a free information pack please contact the Schools Development Officer at:
St. John Ambulance,
1 Grosvenor Crescent,
London SW1X 7EF
Tel: 0171 235 5231 Fax: 0171 235 0796

For schools in Wales, please contact:
St. John Ambulance,
Priory House, Meridian Court,
North Road,
Cardiff CF4 3BL
Tel: 01222 627627 Fax: 01222 627 687

Young Lifesaver

From June 1997, a new and completely updated first aid scheme for schools will be available. Entitled *Young Lifesaver*, this exciting and fun packed video contains all the very latest first aid techniques and comes with comprehensive teachers guide and activity sheets for key stages 2 or 3. The scheme is suitable for children from the age of 7 upwards but is very flexible and can be adapted to suit young people of any age.

St. John Ambulance National Competition for Schools

All schools teaching the Three Cross Award/Young Lifesaver scheme are eligible to enter a team for the competition. Teams consist of three pupils whose skills are put to the test by dealing with a simulated 'real life' accident. Winning teams progress through County and Regional rounds to a National Final in London, usually in July.

ST. JOHN BADGERS

Children between six and ten can become Badgers, the junior members of St. John Ambulance. Badgers meet every week and follow the 'Badger Course in Absolutely Everything', covering subjects such as First Aid, Safety, Games and Hobbies. There are badges and certificates, competitions and outings, and Badgers even have their own magazine, *Badger Buzz*.

ST. JOHN CADETS

As a major national voluntary youth organisation, the St. John Cadets offer much more than a platform for 'out of school' personal development. When trained, Cadets are encouraged to take part in voluntary work in the community, which fosters values of respect, care and responsibility. Often this voluntary work is in the form of First Aid provision with the adult members at public gatherings, sports events and pop concerts. Perhaps less glamorous but equally important is the 'Care in the Community' work, which involves supporting the sick, the elderly and disabled in our communities.

There are over 25,000 St. John Cadets in England and Wales between the ages of 10 to 18. The Cadets are a growing youth organisation with more and more young people benefiting from the wide variety of opportunities provided. In addition to following courses in First Aid and Care, Cadets will learn many other skills on residential weekends specialising in presentation techniques, communication and leadership.

Cadets are also encouraged to obtain the internationally recognised *Duke of Edinburgh's Award* and have the opportunity to participate in a variety of adventurous activities. The prestigious *Grand Priors Award* promotes a range of 'non-first aid' skills - from two way radio communications to baby sitting, and from exploring health and social issues to learning about fire prevention!

There are Badger Sets and Cadet Divisions throughout the UK. Contact the appropriate County Headquarters (addresses on Page 70) for more information, or if you would like to set up a Set or Division in your school.

USEFUL ADDRESSES

St. John Ambulance County Headquarters. Please prefix all addresses with "St John Ambulance"

AVON
The Harry Crook Centre,
Raleigh Road,
Bedminster,
Bristol, BS3 1AP.
(0117) 953 3880

BEDFORDSHIRE
St. John House,
34 St. John's Street,
Bedford, MK42 0DH
(01234) 216200

BERKSHIRE
St. John Centre,
Church Road,
Woodley,
Reading, RG5 4QN
(01734) 442623

BUCKINGHAMSHIRE
Robert Payne Training Centre,
Tindal Road,
Aylesbury,
Bucks, HP20 1HR
(01296) 23886

CAMBRIDGESHIRE
3 Barton Road,
Cambridge, CB3 9JZ
(01223) 355334

CHESHIRE
PO Box 683,
Countess of Chester Hospital
Valley Drive,
Liverpool Road,
Chester, CH1 1FA
(01244) 383407

CLEVELAND
St. John House,
236 Marton Road,
Middlesbrough,
Cleveland, TS4 2EZ
(01642) 218125

CORNWALL
Par Moor Road,
Par,
Cornwall, PL24 2SQ
(01726) 815967

CUMBRIA
Scalegate Road,
Upperby,
Carlisle,
Cumbria, CA2 4PQ
(01228) 28684

DERBYSHIRE
Alma House,
Derby Road,
Chesterfield, S40 2ED
(01246) 200272

DEVON
7-9 Marlborough Court,
Manaton Close,
Matford Business Park,
Exeter,
Devon, EX2 8PF
(01392) 824445

DORSET
St. John House,
1 and 2 Orchard Street,
Dorchester,
Dorset, DT1 1JH,
(01305) 264510

DURHAM
Suite 3,
Townsgate Business Centre,
Littleburn Ind. Estate,
Langley Moor,
Durham City,
Co. Durham, DH7 8HG
(0191) 378 1111

ESSEX
Lancaster House,
140 Mildmay Road,
Chelmsford, CM2 0EB
(01245) 265678

GLOUCESTERSHIRE
St. John House,
67 London Road,
Gloucester, GL1 3HF
(01452) 527227

Gtr MANCHESTER
St. John House,
Egerton Road,
Fallowfield, M14 6XX
(0161) 225 2764

GUERNSEY
Bailiwick Office,
Rohais,
St. Peter Port,
Guernsey GY1 1YN
(01481) 727129

HAMPSHIRE
St. John House,
Worthy Lane,
Winchester, SO23 7AB
(01962) 863366

HERE & WORCS
148 Wylds Lane,
Worcester, WR5 1DN
(01905) 359512

HERTFORDSHIRE
The White House,
Argyle Way,
Stevenage,
Herts, SG1 2AD
(01438) 740044

HUMBERSIDE
Priory House,
Popple St,
Hull, HU9 1LP
(01482) 588564

ISLE of MAN
18 Port-E-Chee Ave,
Douglas, Isle of Man IM2 5E
(01624) 621615

ISLE of WIGHT
12 Manners View,
Dodner Park,
Newport, PO30 5FA
(01983) 822794

JERSEY
Midvale Road,
St. Helier,
Jersey, C.I. JE2 3YR
(01534) 35611

KENT
31 Town Hill,
West Malling
Nr Maidstone,
Kent, ME19 6QL
(01732) 874446

LANCASHIRE
79 Garstang Road,
Fulwood, Preston,
Lancs, PR1 1LD
(01772) 252239

LEICESTERSHIRE
112 Regent Road,
Leicester, LE1 7LT
(01162) 553954

LINCOLNSHIRE
The Cardinal's Hat,
268 High Street,
Lincoln, LN2 1JG
(01522) 523701

LONDON
Edwina Mountbatten House
63 York St,
Marylebone, W1H 1PS
(0171) 258 3456

MERSEYSIDE
PO Box 90,
2 Edgar St,
Liverpool, L69 3RB
(0151) 298 2838

NORFOLK
59 King Street,
Norwich, NR1 1PH
(01603) 621649

NORTHANTS
35 Billing Rd,
Northampton, NN1 5DQ
(01604) 33711

NORTHUMBRIA
St. John House,
Westgate Road,
Newcastle-upon-Tyne,
NE4 9PQ
(0191) 273 7938

N. YORKS
46 Topcliffe Rd,
Thirsk, YO7 1RB
(01845) 522818

NOTTS
561 Valley Road,
Basford,
Nottingham, NG5 1JG
(01159) 784625

OXFORDSHIRE
St. John House,
High Street,
Kidlington,
Oxon OX5 2DN
(01865) 378228

SHROPSHIRE
St. John House,
Priory Road,
Shrewsbury, SY1 1RU
(01743) 231280

SOMERSET
St. John House,
60 Staplegrove Road,
Taunton, TA1 1DH
(01823) 337285

S. & W. YORKS
St. John Hall,
Garden St,
Ravensthorpe,
Dewsbury, WF13 3AR
(01924) 497012

STAFFORDSHIRE
18 Lichfield Road,
Stafford, ST17 4LJ
(01785) 257124

SUFFOLK
St. John House,
30 Samuel Court,
Ipswich, IP4 2EL
(01473) 254005

SURREY
St. John House,
Stocton Close,
Guildford, GU1 1HA
(01483) 450000

SUSSEX
25a Farncombe Road,
Worthing,
West Sussex, BN11 2AY
(01483) 450000

WARWICKSHIRE
National
Agricultural Centre
Stoneleigh,
Kenilworth, CV8 2LZ
(01203) 696521

W. MIDLANDS
Nelson Memorial Hall,
100 Lionel Street,
Birmingham, B3 1DG
(0121) 236 6660

WILTSHIRE
15 High Street,
Devizes,
Wiltshire SN10 1AT
(01380) 728362

WALES
Priory House,
Meridian Court
North Road, Cardiff CF4 3BL
(01222) 627627

N. IRELAND
Erne,
Knockbracken Healthcare Park,
Saintfield Road,
Belfast,
N.Ireland, BT8 8RA
(01232) 799393

SCOTLAND
St. Andrews Ambulance Assoc.,
48 Milton Street,
Glasgow, G4 0HR
(0141) 332 4031

NATIONAL HEADQUARTERS
1 Grosvenor Crescent,
London, SW1X 7EF
(0171) 235 5231

Other useful addresses:

National Asthma Campaign
Providence House
Providence Place
London N1 0NT
Tel: 0171 226 2260

The British Diabetic Association
10 Queen Anne Street
London W1M 0BD
Tel: 0171 323 1531

The British Epilepsy Association
Education Department
Anstey House
40 Hanover Square
Leeds LS3 1BE
Tel: 01532 439393
Helpline: 0800 809030

Health Education Authority
Hamilton House
Mabledon Place
London WC1H 9TX
Tel: 0171 383 3833

SCODA (Standing Conference on
Drug Abuse)
1 Hatton Place
Hatton Garden
London EC1N 8ND
Tel: 0171 430 2341

TACADE (The Advisory Council on
Alcohol and Drug Education)
Publications
No 1 Hulme Place
The Crescent
Salford M5 2QA

INDEX

INDEX

EMERGENCY INDEX